Tired
No More!

David Hazard

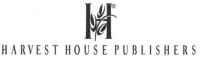

HARVEST HOUSE PUBLISHERS

EUGENE, OREGON

Cover by Left Coast Design, Portland, Oregon

Advisory

Readers are advised to consult with their physician or other medical practitioner before implementing the suggestions that follow.

This book is not intended to take the place of sound medical advice or to treat specific maladies. Neither the author nor the publisher assumes any liability for possible adverse consequences as a result of the information contained herein.

TIRED NO MORE!
Copyright © 2003 by David Hazard
Published by Harvest House Publishers
Eugene, Oregon 97402
www.harvesthousepublishers.com

Library of Congress Cataloging-in-Publication Data

Hazard, David.
    Tired no more! / David Hazard.
        p. cm. — (Healthy body, healthy soul series)
    ISBN 0-7369-1195-2 (pbk.)
    1. Fatigue—Prevention. 2. Health. 3. Dietary supplements. 4. Spirituality. I. Title. II. Series.
    RB150.F37H396 2003
    613—dc21   2003013272

Printed in the United States of America

03   04   05   06   07   08   09   10   11   / BP-MS /   10   9   8   7   6   5   4   3   2   1

Contents

Healthy Body, Healthy Soul

Ancient wisdom tells us we are divinely, intricately "woven together…fearfully and wonderfully made." The sacred scriptures of most major religions tell us that each one of us is a unique marvel of creation—a body and a soul, made to work together in a way that generates a whole-person sort of health and well-being.

Unfortunately, life throws many conditions at us that work to upset the balance we need to achieve and maintain that well-being in body and soul. One of the first signs that something is out of balance is that we lose our personal energy.

Before we're even aware something's wrong…we suffer mental overload…or a conflict in our spirit…we overtax or underwork our body…we *think* we're eating a reasonably nutritious diet but we're really not.

Suddenly, we're dragging. Maybe we've been tired so long we can't remember the last time we felt vital and energetic. We struggle through the day, mentally sluggish, wishing for a nap. Maybe we even slide into chronic illness or depression. We want to quit…go lie down somewhere and just sleep for a long time…but there's no way to escape the demands of life that keep us trudging.

Few things make life feel so tiresome, taxing, and unlivable as having little or no energy.

"Healthy Body, Healthy Soul" is a series of books that takes a whole-person approach to issues affecting our health and wellness. Each book helps you establish personal balance as a way to achieve overall well-being. The goal is to help you create a self-care plan tailored to your personal lifestyle and needs—one you can use whether you're working with a healthcare professional or creating your own plan for re-energizing.

In this book you'll find the best that today's world of natural and complementary healthcare therapies has to offer. From the simple, practical strategies offered here you can create the personalized self-care plan that will give you more energy.

Along with reliable information you'll find encouragement for making these strategies part of your daily life.

Having more energy is the foundation for better total health *and* a more satisfying life. With that in mind, I wish you good health—body and soul!

David Hazard
Founder of *The New Nature Institute*

1

All the Energy You Need

I need *more energy.*" You said that just yesterday…or maybe this morning. And then this radio ad grabbed your attention:

"Feel tired? Dragged-out? Take _____, with its new, patented, super-energizing formula, and have all the energy you need!"

Maybe you've passed by racks of new snack foods in your local grocery or convenience store and read labels that say,

"High-energy food! Now in a delicious-tasting snack [bar, drink, candy]."

These quick pick-me-ups are offered as healthful alternatives to, say, a morning or midday shot of caffeine.

Possibly, you were paging through a magazine and an ad like this jumped out at you:

"Awaken amazing energy…through [this particular exercise or mystical-sounding practice]! Video and audio tapes available."

The promise is, if you learn how to practice this "secret" or "age-old" skill you'll be practically airborne with all that extra energy the cosmos sends your way.

And all you wanted was just to get through the day without feeling so tired.

Unfortunately, anyone who suggests that any single product or practice can give you "all the energy you need" is making an unfounded claim. There is no single "super-energizing formula" or "secret" that can give you boundless energy. And ironically, some of those formulas can actually harm you. Neither can an exercise or

7

meditative technique, by itself, "super-energize" you. Those claims can be misleading…and in the end, frustrating and disappointing.

> *Replenishing your source
> of personal energy begins with a careful,
> mindful approach to life…your life.*

True, certain natural supplements and foods can give you a temporary pick-me-up. So can certain mental and spiritual practices and even physical workouts. In this book you'll learn about many of them—the ones whose effectiveness has been proven over time. But to restore your source of personal energy—a personal reserve, so to speak—you need something more, something better than a quick-fix approach.

More Energy…for Total Well-Being

More personal energy comes as you create a simple plan that uses a safe and natural approach and takes into account the needs of your whole person. This plan should be tailored to your needs, so that it works specifically for *you*. Developing a plan is not hard, however, and it begins with a simple step most of us ignore: paying careful attention to the energy demands in your own life—especially to what *drains* you of energy. Because many of us overlook the obvious, the next chapter will help you complete a simple and revealing "Personal Energy Audit." You may be surprised at what you discover about yourself and what's making you so fatigued.

After you take your audit, the remaining chapters will help you explore safe, natural ways to create more personal energy. You'll discover a wide range of simple and practical strategies for re-boosting personal energy—using a whole-person approach. Because there is no one answer that fits everyone, you can test each of these strategies and discover for yourself the ones that revitalize you. As you find the ones that fit your lifestyle and work for you, that tired-out, dragged-out feeling that makes life dreary will diminish…and you'll start to experience more energy in body, mind, *and* spirit.

Get the Picture?

We human beings are complex creatures. The body itself is made up of many systems. Add to that the complex workings of the mind. And then there are all those deeper issues—that system of beliefs and values that makes us spiritual beings. That leaves us with any number of ways we can become overtaxed…and wake up to find the energy has drained out of us.

Nonetheless, there are some simple principles that are true for all of us. If you observe the following four basic principles you'll bring an overall balance to your life that restores the source of personal energy. As you recognize how these principles relate to you personally you can then begin to focus on the strategies you may need most in order to re-energize.

FOUR PRINCIPLES FOR CREATING MORE PERSONAL ENERGY

Energy Principle #1: All the Energy You Need Comes from "Whole-Person Living"

When most of us have problems we want to fix them quickly…and then get on with our lives just the way we've been living. We want to do the minimum and get the maximum. This unrealistic approach doesn't work…but we keep trying. (Welcome to the human race!)

When we're presented with a challenge to our life and well-being, it's most often because some aspect of our person—body, mind, or spirit—is trying to tell us something. Many times our troubles and symptoms are a warning: *You missed the right road! Go back! Danger ahead!*

Oddly enough, many times the warning is *exactly what we don't want to hear.* Why? Because it's coming from a part of our lives we're afraid to honestly examine. We may think the challenge will be too overwhelming to face. We don't know where the strength or know-how will come from to handle it. We don't have faith that God will be there to help us—giving wisdom and resilience when we need it. (Once again, welcome...)

A persistent lack of energy is a clear and definite warning that some aspect of life is out of balance. But if you take a whole-person approach to your life—instead of hoping quick fixes will do the trick—you will gain in tremendous ways. You'll discover

→ a profound realization of who you are

→ what you need to make life "work for you"—that is, how to live in balance

→ a deeper relationship with the God who gives wisdom and the resilience to overcome challenges

→ more resources to give you increased personal energy

In short, you'll reconnect with a life that's both healthy and full—the life you were meant to live.

By the way, you will find one important theme running through every page of this book, and it comes from the Christian tradition that I honor:

The One who designed us *wants* to energize us—to fill us with joyful vitality. From the brightness of our souls, to the clarity of our minds, to the strength that ignites every muscle fiber in our bodies...we were made to *radiate life.*

If we learn to live in balance and honor the life we've been given, we *will* experience all the energy we need because we were created to be "the light of the world" (Matthew 5:14).

Energy Principle #2:
Carry the Right Load

Many of us *overload* ourselves in one way or another. We work too hard. We eat too much...or just eat too many of the foods that load us down. We may also carry too many unresolved mental or spiritual struggles...whether our own or the burdens of others.

We may feel guilty when we must turn away these burdens, as if it's our duty to be mental or spiritual pack mules. Or maybe we just don't know any other way to approach life than to charge full-speed ahead with a loaded pack on our backs.

We're tired, many of us, because we've exhausted ourselves by carrying burdens in body, mind, or spirit (or all three) that are sapping our vitality.

In the chapters that offer mental and spiritual practices for re-energizing, and in the chapter on nutrition, you'll find great strategies to help you lighten your load.

Energy Principle #3:
Use "Energy Boosters" Sparingly

After the warning not to rely on quick fixes, this principle will seem contradictory—but there are times when we *need* a little energy boost.

The fact is, life's pressures will continue to conspire against us. Just when we've discovered what it means to live in balance...just when we've found the strategies that work for us...we're overwhelmed by demands on our time and energy on the job or at home. Demands that will keep us from eating or taking a break when we need it. We feel the old challenges...or new ones...draining us all over again.

Along with creating a whole-life plan for revitalizing, you will want to put together an "Energy-Boosting Pack" to take along with you during the day. Pay special attention to the strategies in this book—be they mental, spiritual, or physical practices—that can be used anytime and anywhere. Note the energizing snack foods, drinks, and even aromatic oils that can be tucked into a briefcase, purse, or gym bag, and stock up. Also take note of the mental and spiritual strategies you can "take with you," as well as the simple energizing mini-workouts offered, and make them part of your "pack." (This little symbol indicates specially recommended energy boosters.)

You *will* need energy boosters from time to time. Doesn't it simply make sense to carry the *healthiest* and *best* ones along with you?

Energy Principle #4: Having "Enough" Means Living in Sync with Your Energy Flow

There is an ebb and flow to personal energy that's created naturally by our own body chemistry. Many of us live out of sync with these tides.

Most of us come home from a day at work and think, *Why am I so fatigued? I really didn't expend a lot of physical energy today.* The answer is, we're fatigued because we didn't work *enough* physically to boost our metabolism. We didn't place a great enough demand on our bodies to get our biochemistry up and running. Our energy resources are, essentially, untapped.

On the other hand, some of us are burnout cases. Whether because of mental, spiritual, or physical stress, we tend to overtax our body chemistry. We don't know how to stop "with a little left in the tank." Our energy floods out, emptying us.

Then again, many of us pour energy into activities that have no meaning or purpose for us. We work hard at jobs we hate "for the paycheck." We remain in relationships that drag us down because we're unwilling to make changes. We spend a lot of energy keeping up a false front—at home, on the job, at our place of worship—because we're afraid to let other people know what we *really* think or want or believe. Our energy flows into resentment, frustration, and depression, or into creating a false impression.

Just as important, we can be neglectful of our real nutritional and health needs. Maybe we pay little attention to what we eat and drink, or avoid healthcare treatment until and unless we're "really sick." Studies show that few of us get the rest we need, and so on top of personal neglect we're sleep-deprived.

The bottom line here is, we need to rediscover our natural, God-given flow of energy and learn how to live in sync with it.

While you are testing the natural and complementary strategies in this book, my hope is that you'll also be on a journey of self-discovery...and that along the way you'll begin to learn what you need to do to boost your flow of energy so it can power you through even your busiest days.

Take Charge of Your Life... and Begin with Small Changes

Make it a priority to find out how to make your life work in a way that energizes the "outer" physical you...and the "inner" spiritual you, as well.

*But hold on...*the truth is, maybe you picked up this book because you're tired and dragged-out. The thought of revamping your whole life may seem overwhelming. What you *really* want is just a little more energy. *Now.* Well, for that reason the chapters that follow are filled with *dozens of simple, energizing strategies you're after—including small changes you can make that will give you an immediate boost.*

If that's your need—no sweat. But don't give up on the long-term approach. Recognize, though, that the road to every big success is paved with a series of small and significant changes. As the saying goes, "Every great journey begins with just one step."

What's important to remember is this: Any positive change will help you. And even small changes, over time, can add up to *big* change—and that leads to greater health, better balance, and more energy...*all the energy you need!*

2

Why Am I So Tired?

Don't skip this important self-assessment.

I *know* where all my energy is going," says Mike. "I'm getting to bed a little too late. No more staying up to watch the eleven o'clock news." But does Mike *really* know? On second thought, he says, "I guess I'm under some stress at work, too. Do you think that has anything to do with being so tired?"

Bill, an athlete, says he's "100-percent sure I'm tired all the time because I've increased the intensity of my workouts. I don't need to know where all my energy is going. I just want to know how to have *more* energy."

Leslie is also "certain" she knows why her energy level is always so low. "It's hormones. And keeping up with the kids. It just has to be that. Up till now I've always had energy." Her husband smiles and rolls his eyes. "*Or* it could be the fact that you also take on too many projects at the kids' school, in the community, and at church."

Marie and Karl, however, are both genuinely mystified. "We watch our diet," says Marie. "We try to get enough rest. And we're both careful not to take on extra jobs outside of work." "Yeah," Karl adds. "I truly don't know why we're both so tired most of the time."

The Hidden Sources of Your Fatigue

Many of us think we have a good idea why our energy level is low. And because we believe we know where the problem lies, we may even have made certain adjustments. A little more sleep. A little less volunteer work. A few vitamins or supplements. We keep hoping these small changes will restore the energy and joy of living. If they don't, we shrug...and trudge on.

The fact is, most of us are losing energy in ways we do not even recognize. True, we may spot certain factors that contribute to our fatigue. But too often we treat lesser or surface problems while overlooking major things that are draining us of vitality.

The fatigue that plagues us may often be coming from several factors that are at work together, sapping our energy.

Whether we're working with a professional or trying to solve the low-energy puzzle on our own, we'll make greater strides toward boosting our vitality if we take time for a more complete look at ourselves. Amazingly, the various sources of our fatigue will reveal themselves with a bit of careful and honest self-assessment.

You Need an "Audit"

When you think your electric bill is too high, or that it's jumped too much in a given month, you can ask your power company to perform what's called an "energy audit." A technician will come out to your home and take time to assess exactly where all that electricity is going.

When fatigue is robbing us of the life we want, we do well to conduct a "Personal Energy Audit," which this chapter provides—a self-assessment tool to help shed light on where our vitality is going.

On one hand, of course, self-assessment has limitations.

Fatigue can be caused by the fact that your body is not absorbing all the nutrients you need from your food. Or you may be suffering from biochemical imbalance, or from cardiac or respiratory problems, or from the onset of a serious or chronic illness. These things will show up only with the use of special diagnostic skills and equipment. Likewise, mental and emotional conflicts are often best brought to light by professionals who know how to create an understanding environment. Then we feel safe to get past our natural defenses and denials. Then we feel relaxed enough to expose the inner stresses that are draining us of life.

On the other hand, self-assessment can play a very important part in discovering the roots of our personal health problems.

The fact is, even well-trained healthcare professionals can easily miss broader lifestyle conflicts that contribute greatly to our health issues. Many focus intently on their area of specialty. That's what they're trained to do, and it's what they *should* do. But that also means they're combing through scientific details...and may be missing the bigger picture of your whole life. A test for, say, a heart problem or a hormonal imbalance will not reveal other major sources of fatigue lodged in the broader regions of human existence—for instance, emotionally draining relationships, the shock and devastation of grief or loss, or the wrenching stress that overtakes us when we go through a life-passage transition. Shockingly, few healthcare professionals have good training in nutrition—which is so basic to energy and well-being that it's hard to imagine a more glaring instance of negligence on the part of healthcare educators. And any of these broader factors can quickly deplete us.

Give Yourself This Good Gift

The bottom line is this: You are the person who stands on the front lines of your own life. When it comes to your well-being, no one stands to lose more by not acting than you...or to gain more by taking a step back and looking at the broader scope of your whole life.

You are the best person to begin the total "energy audit" and determine what's draining the vitality out of you. What you discover about yourself and your lifestyle will be valuable information, whether you use this knowledge to create a self-care plan or decide to seek help from a caring professional.

A PERSONAL ENERGY AUDIT

What follows is a self-test that can help you
focus on aspects of your life that may require care and attention.
Take time to carefully consider each of the following
areas where you may be draining yourself of energy.

Audit Area #1:
Using Too Much Mental Energy

Some of us are "linear thinkers," meaning that we generally need to be left alone to concentrate on one thing at a time, thank you.

Others can handle a variety of mental activities all at once. We can talk on the phone...*and* check e-mail...*and* work on a dinner recipe...*and* handle distractions from our kids...Or we can keep one major lobe of our brain in an intense office meeting...*while* mentally composing a report we need to finish by the end of the day.

Expending mental energy can be very tiring, even if you believe you thrive on chaos. Why? Because all that mental focus has a collateral effect on our physical body. As our thoughts intensify, our muscles tense up, our heart beats faster, and breathing gets shallow. We may come to the end of a workday and say, "All I did was sit at a computer working on reports today...but I'm *exhausted*."

The tiredness you and I feel after a mentally challenging day is *real* fatigue. The problem is, we may be used to mental multitasking. The stresses we carry inside our heads may actually feel "normal" to us by now. We may need to step back just to recognize how our mental load is wiping us out.

Consider the following, and see if any of these conditions have become a mental drain on your energy. Check the conditions that apply to you, and fill in the blanks.

_____ **Mental multitasking.** Do too many things demand your attention all at once? Do you find yourself in the middle of one thought...or one action...only to realize you've lost your concentration and your mind is somewhere else? Or that you've completely forgotten what you were about to do or say?

When I am (where?)_____ I find myself being distracted by (what?)_____ .

_____ **Mental confusion.** In the past you were a shining example of clear thinking. Now, however, you lose your train of thought or realize you're rambling when you speak. These are signs of mental energy overload. You are moving toward the breaking point.

I lose my train of thought...or wonder what I was about to do or say...or forget crucial details like important appointments (when?)

_____

_____ .

_____ **Mental breaking point.** When mental stress reaches overload you can expect to experience a breakdown in your normal decorum. Logic goes out the window and emotions flood in. Frustration and feeling overwhelmed can trigger sudden floods of emotions, from anger to tears, to despair and desperation. You are expending way too much energy trying to hold yourself together.

*Mentally, I hit my breaking point (how often?)*_____

*when I am overloaded mentally by (what or who?)*_____

_____ .

Audit Area #2:
Using Too Much Spiritual Energy

For the purposes of this book, we're defining "spirit" as that part of us that *holds our deepest values*. It's the part of us that *maintains our sense of where we stand in relationship toward our selves, other people, and God.*

When all's right in this deepest aspect of our being we feel buoyant and energetic, and there is a spring in our step. But when something in our life has us at odds with our own values we begin to expend energy on spiritual stress. We work hard to avoid, ignore, deny, or justify what we're doing. Likewise, when we're at odds with our self, with someone we value, or with God, our spirit feels stressed or weighed down.

Most intense of all, we can experience a collapse of our whole belief system. All our energy can seem to rush out...leaving us listless, feeling "flat" or "dead."

Do any of the following conditions apply to you?

_____ **Spiritual tension.** Our values give life meaning and purpose. Values are like the thread that holds together body and soul. When we experience two of our values being at odds with one another, a deep-soul tension is created. Our belief that it's good to be honest may war against our belief that saying the truth will hurt someone. Our belief that we should be loyal to our spouse and to family ties may be wrestling with a pull to fulfill personal desires in a new relationship. We expend a lot of energy trying to "keep things under control."

Often, too, many of us judge or suppress our spiritual conflicts. We think we can ignore them away, or we just pretend we're "beyond" this kind of struggle. A lot of daytime energy goes into denial and suppression...and we wake up exhausted after nights of troubled dreams and fitful sleep.

Conflict with ourselves, with another person, or with God can also demand a huge expense of spiritual energy. Perhaps we're angry or hateful or punishing toward ourselves for some perceived lack or failure. Maybe we harbor anger or bitterness toward ourselves. Maybe our disappointment or anger with God is too scary to voice out loud...or even admit. Even more energy goes into self-recrimination...criticizing and blaming others...or being stuck with unexpressed negative feelings toward God.

*I am experiencing conflict between (which spiritual values?)*_____

_____ .

*I am experiencing conflicting feelings toward (whom?)*_____

because _____ .

_____ **Spiritual breakdown.** When we experience a deep-soul-level connection with another person or group, or with an important support system (family, friends, spiritual community) we feel energetic and flooded with life. But when a relationship is breaking down we can also begin to experience it as a physical letdown.

*I have experienced a shake-up in, or break with, my past beliefs about (what?)*_____

_____ .

*I feel cut off from (whom?)*_____

because _____ .

_____ **Spiritual disconnect.** Maybe you've never really connected with any beliefs that have inspired you or ignited a passion to live for anything beyond your immediate needs, wants, or comforts. Life just seems "flat."

Or maybe you've been through an experience that crushed your beliefs or deepest hopes. Your sense of connection to spiritual realities has snapped, and the pilot light of your spiritual zeal has gone out. Sometimes you just feel dead inside.

*I don't have any strong beliefs or spiritual passions because*_____

_____ .

*I used to have strong beliefs, but I gave them up when*_____

_____ .

Audit Area #3:
Using Too Much Energy
Maintaining Relationships

Another of the areas of life that drains our energy—an area most of us are blind to—is in our relationships. While it's obvious when the kids are "running you ragged" or your parent, spouse, or boss is a "demanding taskmaster," certain aspects of relationships can drain us of mental, spiritual, or physical energy…and we may not be all that aware of it.

_____**Responding to pressure or demands.** Sometimes people press us…and we get used to giving in. The kids demand this. The boss yells for that. We keep giving in, even when the pressure has gotten really old and we're overtaxed. Or…maybe we really do hold the line. We keep saying no and resisting certain people's constant pressure. But the energy of resisting is wearing us down inside and

out. Either way, relationships that pressure us leave us feeling overworked and fatigued.

*I feel pressured by (whom?)*_____
(and how often?) _____ .

_____**Everybody's "slave."** You are everybody's "go-to" guy or girl—
maybe at home, maybe at work. Maybe both. You need to off-load
some duties but haven't spoken up yet.

Sometimes we stay stuck in the "slave" mode because we tell ourselves it's easier to do it ourselves than train someone else to do what
we do. We make the beds because "the kids don't know how to do it
right." Or we balance the checkbooks, write all the bills, and handle
all the home repairs because "the little woman isn't good at these
things."

It's also possible we even secretly *like* having everybody need us.
It makes our place in their hearts, or in their organization, feel more
secure. But the price we pay for feeling "valued" is exhaustion.

Bottom line: We overperform…and allow other people to underperform…and we're tired.

I am overworking in my relationship (with whom?) _____ *by*
doing (what?) _____ *when they can*
do this themselves.

_____**The great peacekeeper, or interpreter.** In some relationships
we become the go-between. We "interpret" one friend's thoughtless
or cold comments to another. We put a softer "spin" on something
harsh our spouse said to our child. We keep co-workers focused and
moving ahead on projects when their squabbling threatens to bog
down work at the office. Instead of learning how to help people work
out their differences themselves, those of us who are peacekeepers or
interpreters spend an enormous amount of physical and mental
energy trying to keep others' relationships flowing.

I spend a lot of time and energy being a peacekeeper, the interpreter
between (who?) in order to keep (what process or relationship?)
_____ *running smoothly.*

_____ **Holding the relationship together.** Sometimes, too, we just put too much energy into maintaining a relationship that's not balanced. We do all the calling, e-mailing, and setting up dates. Everything is left to us.

I am putting out a lot of energy to maintain a relationship with (whom?)_____ because I am afraid that if I don't (what will happen?) _____ .

Audit Area #4:
Using Too Much Physical Energy

It might seem obvious when we're expending too much physical energy and running our tanks dry. And for some of us that's true. We know what we're doing. But that's not necessarily true for all of us.

Many of us are programmed to push too hard, or to fill our schedules with too many tasks. We can overestimate our strength and level of endurance—so the workaholic, the driven athlete, and the supermom are all at risk here. We may feel guilty if we don't fall into bed exhausted every night, or if we haven't totally burned out our muscles during a workout. Unfortunately, those of us who push too hard also devalue sleep and relaxation…and usually don't have a clue how much time it really takes for our body to recover after physical exertion. (Hint: *a lot.*)

Do any of the following conditions apply to you?

_____ **Physical overwork.** When we expend too much physical energy—whether at work or at "play"—we can exhaust all the major systems of our bodies. We create conditions that keep us chronically fatigued. Our mood darkens, our interest in sex wanes. We're headachy, cranky, and hard to live with. We also deplete our immune system, opening ourselves to any serious health conditions to which we may be genetically predisposed and also to serious pathogens from the environment. In short, we wipe out our body's natural defenses.

I do not have enough energy to get through my work day without feeling fatigued…sometimes even exhausted…and this occurs (how often?) _____ .

I sometimes doze off, or want to nap, in the middle of my workday, and this happens (how often?) _____ .

I sometimes work myself to exhaustion doing (what job or task?) _____ .

I experience colds, headaches, and other symptoms of illness (how often?) _____ *, and suspect my immune system may be depleted.*

_____ **Underresting.** Studies have proven that a majority of adults in our culture are sleep-deprived. Some of us just can't or won't take a day off. We even fill our "vacations" with activity. Resting may seem like "a waste of time" or even make us feel guilty.

I sleep for _____ hours and still wake up feeling tired or even exhausted.

I am unable to complete or engage in physical workouts (how often?) _____ *because I feel too tired.*

I take days off to rest and recover (how often?) _____ *, and I take longer vacations to rest and renew myself (how often?)* _____
_____ .

Audit Area #5:
Using Not Enough *Energy*

"I really don't get it," says Denise. "I work at a desk all day and don't expend that much energy. Why am I so wiped out at the end of a day?"

Terry echoes her complaint. "I sleep a *lot.* And my wife complains that I'm a 'couch potato' because I lie around watching sports on TV. It doesn't make sense that I have no energy…but I just don't."

As damaging as it is to overwork and use too much energy…not using enough energy can also leave us feeling fatigued. The reason is simple: When you rest *too much* you rarely kick your metabolism into a higher gear. Digestion slows, and all the rest of your biochemistry goes into slow motion as well. While the healthcare community recommends we get *at least* 30 minutes of good aerobic exercise three times a week, some of us rarely hit that minimum standard. The result is a kind of restless or sluggish fatigue.

How would you answer these questions?

I lead a very sedentary or "laid-back" kind of life, and I engage in strenuous physical work or exercise only (how often?) _____ .

My favorite pastimes include (which sports or kinds of exercise?) _____ , *and*

(which non-athletic hobbies, interests, or escapes?) _____

_____ .

I normally sleep more than eight or nine hours a night, sometimes (how many hours per day, including naps?) _____ .

Audit Area #6:
Eating an Unbalanced Diet

Some of us do not get the right balance of nutrients we need to energize our bodies. This can be true for several reasons.

_____ **Unbalanced eating.** Maybe we eat too much meat, and our body is struggling and overtaxed trying to digest all that protein. Or we eat too few complex carbohydrates—the fruits and vegetables; and we ride the sugar roller coaster that wreaks havoc on our bodies because we eat too many simple carbs: the breads, pastas, grains. Or our vegetarian diet is deficient in important nutrients...With today's overmarketing of supplements, some of us also pop nutritional supplements when we might be better off getting our energy from whole foods.

I hate, or eat very little (protein? complex carbs?) _____ .

I love, or eat a lot of (protein, complex carbs?) _____ .

I use supplements, not just to augment *my nutritional needs but to* meet *my nutritional needs (how often?)* _____ .

_____ **Overeating.** Then there are those of us who simply overeat. We eat till we're full…and overfull…to satisfy our need for the "comfortable feeling" of a full tummy…or because we just love flavorful foods. All this overstuffing drains us. It draws the blood from our extremities as our body struggles to digest the load we've eaten. And our other bodily systems are drained as our biochemistry shifts, trying to work with the overabundance of inflooding nutrients. And then there's the issue of carrying around extra weight. Ironically, eating more gives us less energy.

I eat until I feel too full (how often?) _____ .

I overeat because (what's your reason?) _____

_____ .

_____ **Undereating.** Many more of us today *undereat.* Maybe we have problems with our own body image, or maybe we're in a sport or profession that demands we stay "slim." More and more of us are just too crazily busy to slow down and eat right. We are just not getting enough nutrients to keep our bodies functioning at a healthy and energized level. Essentially, we're starving and straining our bodies.

Moreover, the dieting industry has also done a number on us when it comes to "fat." We *need* certain beneficial fats in order for our body to function well and feel energized. Rather than eating fat in the right balance, too many people declare war on all dietary fat…then wonder why they're unhealthy and fatigued.

I have a problem with my body image because I do not like the appearance of my (what aspect of your body?) _____ .

I eat too little because I am trying to maintain a certain weight or slim appearance for (what reason?) _____ .

When it comes to dietary fat, I eat (a lot? very little? virtually none?)

_____ .

3

More Mental Energy!

I get to the middle of my workday, and I'm so mentally fatigued I can hardly think straight. And there are still important client meetings ahead."

"Some evenings my brain is drained. I'm so mentally wiped out I can't think of what to make for dinner."

"My *mind* feels tired. Is that even possible?"

Yes—mental fatigue is possible.

More importantly, there is something you can do to stop mental exhaustion and have the mental energy you need.

What Do You Think?

As a person thinks...so is he. That piece of ancient wisdom from the Bible points to an important practical insight: *How we think affects every aspect of the way we live.*

Perhaps you're aware your mental attitude has the power to affect your health and well-being. People who carry worry, fear, and anger, and people who stress out much of the time, cause their immune systems to operate at a very low level. So they are less able to prevent sickness and disease. Their sleep and digestion are also less than optimal. Therefore, their bodies are less able to restore and repair themselves. Eventually, the result is illness or a serious physical injury. The psychosomatic factor that triggers illness is widely documented.

But are you aware that your mental attitude also has a profound impact on your store of personal energy?

Perhaps you've never thought of it this way, but something as seemingly passive as thinking requires *real energy*. If you've ever had electrical-impulse sensors attached to your head to track the function of your brain waves, you know there is indeed live voltage circulating inside your skull. The fact is, the *kind* and *amount* of mental energy we expend has a major effect on our health and well-being.

Long before illness or injury makes it obvious that our approach to life needs to change, we can be misusing mental energy in ways that harm us. True, all of us have negative or unpleasant thoughts from time to time. But for some of us, living in a negative mental state is habitual. And because it's habitual, it erodes our health. No wonder we are drained of energy.

If we're smart—if we want more energy—we'll give ourselves some "TLC."

In this chapter, we'll look for signs that tell us we're using our mental energy in unhealthy ways. Then we'll look at strategies we can use to change energy-depleting thought patterns and mental habits and find more healthful ways to use our minds.

Are You In the (+) or (–) Zone?

Below are lists describing some of the more intense mental states we can experience. To be sure, most of us experience some of these at one time or another. But are any of these symptoms or tendencies characteristic of your *usual* mental state? Or do you experience swings from one state to another—from positive to negative, or negative to positive?

(—)	(+)
___ *sluggish thinking*	___ *thoughts that race or go into "overdrive"*
___ *confused thinking*	___ *rigid thinking*
___ *imprecise, lax thinking*	___ *being obsessive about "rule keeping"*
___ *poor memory*	___ *being stuck on details*
___ *sad or depressive thoughts*	___ *euphoric thoughts*

___ *thoughts about being "trapped"*	___ *thoughts of being "limitless"*
___ *self-destructive thoughts*	___ *thoughts of being indestructible*
___ *obsessive or intrusive thoughts*	___ *thoughts interrupted by emotional "highs"*

Negative-zone thinking has the effect on your inner being that carrying heavy weights has on your physical body. It rapidly depletes your energy and leaves you drained and tired. Too many of us handle negative thinking by sleeping or indulging in other low-energy escapes. Sometimes we medicate the unpleasant sensations generated by negative thinking with food, alcohol, or drugs.

If your mental energy is spent mostly in the *negative zone,* you may need to seek the support of a caring professional. In fact, you may need the help of a counselor or clergyman to address underlying life issues—ones that are difficult for any one of us to face on our own. Having an outside voice that is coming from a positive, supportive place can be the wonderful, healing, and freeing experience we need to help turn things around.

Even if your mental energy is mostly spent in the *positive zone,* it may surprise you to learn that you can benefit from some strategies for mental balancing. Some of us get locked into a kind of mental exhilaration that is highly charged and gives us the energy of an engine firing on 72 pistons. But the truth is, the mental high we experience is only temporary. We burn ourselves out. (We probably burn other people out, too.)

For some of us, this supercharged state needs to be balanced out so our energy can be distributed more evenly over the span of a day. For others, the near-euphoric state we sometimes experience may be a sign that professional advice is needed to help us achieve better mental balance.

Many of us who are "type A's," however, are simply "addicted" to our own adrenaline. We love reaching the euphoria-like state that carrying a huge mental load gives us. And so we load…and over-load…our brains (and our lives) with projects and details the way a caffeine addict overloads on morning coffee. We may think of it as "mental multitasking," and we may pride ourselves on being capable of handling vast "gigabytes" of information all at once.

But the simple fact is, we are not computers. The mental "burn" we push to achieve drains our physiology in much the same way as the physical burn we push for in weight training drains our muscles of energy. Without balance, without giving ourselves time to ease off and recover, we eventually push ourselves to exhaustion…and even illness.

More Mental Energy!

There is a simple rule in the creation of every type of personal energy. *It takes energy to make energy.* And there is a second rule. *Energy serves us best when it's spent carefully over a period of time.*

Most of us *expend* mental energy—but we don't know how to energize our thinking in the first place, and we don't know how to re-energize when we're mentally fatigued and depleted.

Too, some of us are energy hoarders. We don't put out much effort, and we're left with a lot of potential but unused energy. Then there are those of us who go for broke and blow all our energy at once…then we're burned out.

What follows are simple, natural strategies you can use to help you create more mental energy *and* use it wisely…and thus have all the energy you need.

THE MORE MENTAL ENERGY STRATEGIES

Strategy #1:
Lose the Mental Clutter

Many of us go through life collecting mental "clutter." This can include

→ *"problems"*—that is, potential or imagined problems we've created, or problems for which we are not part of the solution

→ *other people's responsibilities*

→ *mental conversations*—in particular, ones we never actually have with others

→ *details of life*—ones that are important but remain unorganized

Think of your brain as a business office. A business office functions best when it is focused on its most important priorities—and is well-organized to support those priorities. When the employees lose their focus, when the filing system is a jumble, there is confusion, stress…and major expense of energy is needed to keep any business flowing at all. It's the same with your mind: A lack of priority focus and lack of organization to support what's important causes mental stress…resulting in fatigue.

Do This:

Step 1: Set your priorities. No—this is not your "to-do list." That has probably driven you to exhaustion long enough. Figuring out what priority #1 is, is not a luxury. It's an essential. And it's like setting in place a solid foundation on which all your other choices can be made.

Take time to answer these questions:

- **What is the one most important thing I can do today in each of the most important areas of my life?**
- **Whose work—or worries—am I taking on that needs to be handed back to them?**

A word about setting priorities: They will change over time. So take time once a month to check in with your life to see if you need to reprioritize. But *do* set priorities in place for now.

Step 2: Use a magic organizer. Okay, so there's no such thing as a "magic" organizer—but they work like magic if you use them. A simple, inexpensive day planner not only helps you schedule your top priorities, it also helps you be realistic about how much you can actually get done. And it can help you relax and not worry about "remembering" some important detail of your day. It's in the organizer!

Again, flexibility is important. You don't want to be enslaved by what your organizer says—but remember, your mental fatigue is *not* setting good boundaries for your head to follow.

A word about scheduling: Think in terms of scheduling for a week, not just a single day. Most of us try to jam too much into one day. When it doesn't get done, or when it does get done but we're still stressed and fatigued, we tend to say, "This doesn't help at all."

But using an organizer does work...*if you're realistic about the way to work with it.*

Step 3: Get rid of the clutter! We started out talking about mental clutter, such as problems we can do nothing about—and all we've been talking about so far is setting our top priorities and scheduling ourselves. That's right. That's because it's important to have a life you can wholeheartedly say *yes* to...so we can know what we need to say *no* to. Knowing what's most important to you and building your life around it is one of the healthiest things you can do for your mental well-being.

But now comes another challenge—especially for some of us. Give jobs, duties, tasks, and worries back to the people they belong to. Ask yourself the following:

- **Who does this problem *most* directly affect? Who *needs* to handle this task or responsibility?** If your answer is not "me," then someone else is siphoning off your mental energy and getting a free ride. (No wonder you're mentally tired. You've been thinking for two...or perhaps even more!)

- **Clearly communicate to the other person that you are no longer willing, or able, to carry their share of the load.** You don't have to be mean—just be clear. And also strong. Fear can be a big deterrent here. What if they're angry? What if they insist they can't? What if it's our boss—and we might lose our job? The real question is this: *What is your mental well-being worth to you?*

- **Have your "deflector shield" ready.** If and when the other party tries to hand you back the clutter of their life...or if you're in the bad habit of care-taking other people's lives... prepare yourself with a list of good reasons why overloading your head again is a bad idea. Start with "...because I was mentally exhausted and didn't like my life when I did this before."

Step 4: Be honest about the "downtime" you spend. So you want a latte and a catch-up chat with a friend. Pencil it in. Just be firm when it's time to move on. Sometimes, if we're honest, our own little "escapes" cause our day to jam up, and then our stressed-out attempts to catch up wipe out any mental-energy gains we've made.

Strategy #2: Indulge Yourself in the Best "Brain Food"

Maybe you've heard that certain foods—fish, for instance—are good "brain food." There's some truth to that, and in a later chapter we'll see why some foods do energize you better than others.

But thoughts can be like food, as well. Some thoughts get you excited. Others bring you down and leave you feeling wiped out.

When was the last time you felt mentally stimulated—enthusiastic and full of energy? What were you thinking that made you feel that way? Do you know where *your* mental energy comes from? What recharges your thought processes and gets you excited? What makes your thoughts soar like a bird on the wing or burn through the cosmos like a blazing comet?

Mental energy comes, in part, from the kinds of thoughts you think. For that reason, we can benefit greatly if we learn to think of thoughts as brain food. Some thoughts weigh us down and make us sluggish...while others lift us up and give us energy.

Do This:

Step 1: "Eat" for inspiration. The Bible offers some great advice: "Whatsoever things are true...pure...lovely...think on these things." What are you thinking when you begin your day? When your head's not occupied with your priorities, what kind of thoughts occupy your mind throughout the day? To "feed" your mind something uplifting and inspiring,

- **bookend your days with inspirational reading.** Morning or evening or both, feed a positive tone into your waking and sleeping by reading something inspirational.

- **carry inspirational "snack food."** Most days run us up against cranky kids, complaining co-workers, belligerent drivers…not to mention the naturally negative tendencies some of us fight. To counter these wearying forces, it helps to carry small doses of inspiration in the form of

  ~ *simple positive statements you create to reinforce a positive philosophy about life.* These may be original ideas of your own, or wise and positive statements you've picked up along the way. Write them on reminder cards if necessary.

  ~ *inspiring messages.* Whether you prefer uplifting music or positive teachings, tapes or CDs work well while running errands or commuting. Check out your library or your favorite author's Web site.

Step 2: Add a dash of humor. Giving yourself a good laugh every day goes a *long* way toward releasing mental heaviness and increasing mental energy. That's because laughter triggers the body's relaxation response, releasing the nonstress and healing hormones, and we experience this as a good, natural "high." To your inspirational reading and listening list add

  ~ *humorous books, tapes, or CDs* from your favorite comedian or humorist.

The next strategy is equally important…

Strategy #3: Try a Mental "Fast"

Eating the right mental "food" is one part of energizing our brain. Eliminating the kind of thinking that makes us sluggish and heavy is just as important. Negative thoughts, upsetting thoughts, ugly thoughts…these weigh us down and wear us out mentally. We can benefit from regularly cleansing our thoughts by going on a mental "fast."

Do This:

Step 1: Identify the energy-draining "mind food" that needs to be eliminated.

- **Variation 1: Fast from negative talking.** Listen to your own conversations. How often do negative, critical, sarcastic, bitter, or fearful words come out of your mouth? For just one day, refrain from indulging in any negative talk.

- **Variation 2: Fast from negative self-talk.** Listen to your own "internal monologue." That's the voice, or collection of voices, always running *behind* your thoughts. The voices that are constantly telling you what to think and how to feel about what you're experiencing or who you are.

  Some of us are fed by mostly positive internal monologues. A friendship ends and we tell ourselves, "Gee, that's too bad. But life changes and people change. Soon I'll meet new people." Others of us feed ourselves a negative-on-negative self-talk that grinds us down. "He dumped you. That's because you're a loser and you always do something to ruin a good friendship."

- **Variation 3: Fast from the media.** Ads are there to make you feel discontented with what you have and make you want something new. The news is there to scare the pants off you. The shows are there to keep your mind racing or distracted and your adrenaline pumping. Most of it is mentally wearisome (not to mention, a waste of time).

Step 2: For one day, eliminate this particular "mind food." Write a note to yourself if you have to, but find a way to remind yourself, "I'm not going to wear myself out by indulging in mental junk food."

THIS WORKS LIKE A MIRACLE!

～

There is a fast and simple way to re-energize your head when mental fatigue is draining your circuits. *Learn to shift your focus.*

When we're tired out mentally, it's usually because our mind is intensely occupied with too much—that is, too much detail, or too much stressful, heavy, or "down" thinking. When we become overfocused, our breathing will become shallow, too. Not only are we taxing our brain's biochemistry, we're depriving our brain of oxygen (not to mention what mental stress triggers in the rest of our body).

You can boost yourself back to a more energized mental state by doing this:

Step 1: Put it on the shelf. Notice the thing that is gripping your attention with such intensity. Notice that your eyes are narrow-focused, like "zoom lenses." Imagine you're able to set the thing that has your attention—even if it's a plaguing memory or thought—"on a shelf in the back of your head" for a little while.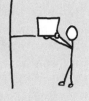

Step 2: Let your mind wander free. Relax your eyes and let them re-train themselves on "distance"—on the horizon or the sky. If you're indoors, let them drift up to a point high on the wall. Feel your focus broaden and your breathing relax and deepen.

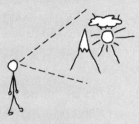

If those demanding thoughts come back, "return them to the shelf."

The tranquillity this simple strategy brings will boost your mind with a *restful but alert* kind of energy. And you can use it virtually anytime and anywhere stressful thinking starts draining your head.

Strategy #4:
Mental Catalysts

When we experience mental sluggishness it's often due to "stuck thinking." We've worn a rut and now we're stuck in it, thinking the same dull dry thoughts over and over. This is like chewing on a piece of food long after the nutrients have been gotten out of it.

New thoughts are "catalytic" in that they literally spark the flow of positive mental energy. Sometimes when we're stuck in mental doldrums, it may seem like we need to revamp our whole life. Many times, though, what we need is simply a fresh perspective and new pursuits.

Do This:

Variation #1: Act on a dream...even if it's taking just a baby step. What's one dream you haven't acted on? To create something? Start a business? Travel? Run a marathon? Maybe you're stuck in a mental rut because you think you can't act on your dream right now...or because you don't have the skill to do it...and all that subliminal frustration is wearing you down.

You need to ask yourself: What's one step *I can take toward my dream?* Most of us make the same big mistake: Because we can't see how we're going to be able to complete the journey, we don't take the first steps. So we leave ourselves stuck in mental doldrums.

People who keep their lives moving...one step at a time...know that a big key to mental energy is keeping themselves out on an edge where their creative-thinking and problem-solving skills are being challenged.

Variation #2: Do something completely new...something that's "not you." Maybe you've accomplished all your big dreams...or you're not a "big dream" kind of person. Okay. Trying something that's just *not you* can be wonderfully mentally stimulating.

You say you're not creative? Try a course in painting or sculpting, or learn to play a musical instrument. Not mechanically inclined? Try small-engine or bike repair. Not athletic? Take an aerobics or beginning fitness class…or get trained for a marathon. So you burn water? A creative cooking class is just the thing. Confirmed homebody? Try an adventure trip to some exciting place you've never visited.

Do you have a social, political, or spiritual stand you hold to strongly? Read something new and challenging from those who oppose your position.

The point is to exercise your mind in brand-new ways. And moving toward the very thing you'd "never" do will provide a wonderful, catalytic spark to your mind…and your life!

IS DEPRESSION BLOCKING YOUR VITAL ENERGIES?

∾

One major cause for mental flatness is depression. Depression is like a logjam in the river of your vitality.

Many of us don't like to admit we're depressed. That goes against our image of ourselves as competent adults who can handle anything, thank you very much. Some of us don't even recognize we're in depression. We are functionally depressed—meaning that we function as if everything's normal when underneath it all we have negative feelings and thoughts.

Depression has many causes. One is repressing, ignoring, or denying thoughts and emotions that are so unpleasant we don't want to meet them head-on. Another is brain chemistry that is out of balance. Bodily sickness, illness, or injury, poor nutrition, or habitual inactivity can cause our body chemistry to sink to a low level of action…creating a "body-based" depression.

If you are depressed, be honest with yourself and get attention for this serious condition. To leave your depression untreated is to slowly lose the gift of life you've been given and, in its place, accept slow death.

Seek out a professional who can help you…and don't stop until you find one who will do more than write a prescription for antidepressants. Find the source of your depression…and get your vitality flowing again.

Strategy #5: Lighten "Emotionally Charged" Thinking

Has anyone ever told you that you're "high-strung"? Or that you can "make a mountain out of a molehill"?

Some of us burn ourselves out mentally...and we burn out other people, too...because our thinking is emotionally charged much of the time. That is, almost every thought has an emotion attached to it—whether it's fear, worry, anger, or sky-high enthusiasm.

Emotions are charged with energy. And some of us drain our vitality because we don't know how to tone down emotionally charged thinking and think in a relaxed mode. Emotions, of course, have a place in our thinking. When we deny them we become depressed and sick. (See sidebar on page 38.) But we can have more mental energy if we learn how to prevent our emotions from over-charging our thoughts and draining our vitality.

Do This:

Step 1: Picture your thoughts as a broad stream. Your mind is a constant flow of thought. Some of it is logical, factual. ("It's sunny today.")

Step 2: Picture the smaller feeder streams of emotion that feed into your thoughts. Imagine *sadness* as its own feeder stream...and *worry*...and *depression*...and *anger*. How many of these regularly feed into your thoughts? ("Yeah, it's sunny...and that just makes me think about how sad I am I have no one to share this great day with.")

Some feeder streams are also full of negative charge. ("Sunny days stink. The light just gives me a headache.")

Step 3: Practice "neutrally charged" thinking. Isolate the bare facts within your thought stream again. Facts themselves are neutrally charged—until we add the emotional charge to them.

Make a simple statement of fact. ("It's a sunny day.") It may take some practice to quiet the feeder steams of emotion and just relax.

The point is to return to basic reality…free of the charged, emotional overlay.

Step 4: Be creative. Ask yourself, "What's the most creative, positive thing I can do, given the facts as they are?" Let's say you don't have someone to share the day with—but what can *you* do that would add joy or satisfaction to the day anyway?

Yes, you will need time and space to let your emotions be what they are. To ignore feelings for very long is to set yourself up for poor health and relational disasters.

But those of us who are emotionally high-pitched need a break from our own exhausting feelings. By practicing this strategy we can retrieve a great deal of the energy emotions burn up and use it in more constructive ways.

Strategy #6: Create a Quiet Place "Inside"

Most of us burn up a lot of mental energy—and physical energy, too—in *stress thinking*. We feel bombarded by noise, schedules, other people's demands. We take on, or accept, additional tasks on top of the ones we already can't handle. By the end of the day we're so tired it's hard to remember our own names.

Not only do we experience exhaustion from stress thinking, but stress is one of the leading causes of many major, debilitating illnesses. Medical studies reveal that more than half of the people suffering from life-threatening conditions—including cancer, heart disease, and immune disorders—have not learned how to manage stress.

But you can. If you need to de-stress, you can do so any time, anywhere, by using this simple strategy.

Do This:

Step 1: Find a quiet spot where you can be alone. This can be indoors, perhaps in a chair by a sunny window. Or outdoors in a quiet park or other natural setting. Chapels, churches, and other places of worship work well, too.

Step 2: Focus on your breathing. Let it become calm and regular. Whether you sit, kneel, or stroll, fix your attention on your breath as it moves in and out through your nostrils. Be relaxed so that your breath can settle into a tidal rhythm, like ocean surf. Breathe deeply enough to fill your lungs, but don't force your breathing.

Step 3: Don't fight with your thoughts. Keep turning your focus to your breathing. Thoughts will try to swarm you like pesky gnats. Major issues that demand attention will rise in your thinking. This is not the time for them…but you also can't stop them by brute force. (The more you fight them the more focused on them you become.) Instead, every time you notice yourself thinking, gently turn your attention back to your breathing.

Continue this practice for several minutes. Build up to longer periods over time.

Step 4: Notice the quiet *behind* the quiet. Eventually, you'll notice that most quiet atmospheres are not that quiet. Little noises are everywhere. But if you pay attention to your breathing, eventually you'll notice an inner quietness—accompanied by a deep sense of peace—forming inside you.

Welcome to an interior place of peace…and a restfulness that is amazingly re-energizing! With practice you will be able to use this strategy even in the midst of busy and pressured circumstances. Instead of depleting your energy in stress thinking, you'll be able to relax and re-energize your mind *and* body.

In Closing

Mental fatigue is one way our inner energy is drained. Tiredness at a deeper level—in our spirit—is another. In the next chapter, we'll look at the ways we become depleted in spirit, and strategies to re-energize at this deeper level of our being.

IS IT ANXIETY...OR OBSESSION?

∽

Everyone experiences common anxiety. Many people are perfectionistic and a bit obsessive about certain things. But for some, anxiety can cross the line and become life-limiting, mentally draining them of energy.

Today, the healthcare community recognizes that certain levels of anxiety are, in fact, disorders. And the great news is, they can be treated.

Do you suffer from any of the following?

~ *intrusive thoughts that disrupt your regular thought stream*

~ *feeling compelled to perform certain personal "rituals" to relieve anxious feelings*

~ *needing to constantly wash or clean because you sense contamination*

~ *overwhelming anxiety or fears that limit what you can do, where you can go, what you can touch*

~ *experiencing sudden, intense panics*

~ *having a list of words, sounds, thoughts, or objects that are "bad"*

~ *feeling compelled to make facial or other bodily movements*

~ *experiencing intense or irrational fears about certain objects or places*

This is only a partial list of conditions that fall under the category of anxiety and anxiety disorders. If you have any of these symptoms or others like them, you know how energy draining they are.

Today, make the commitment to retrieve the energy that's being lost to anxiety by finding a healthcare professional who knows how to treat debilitating anxiety and its related disorders. (You may also benefit from some of the strategies recommended in *Overcoming Anxiety*...another book in the Healthy Body, Healthy Soul series.)

4

More Spirited!

Many people who have been diagnosed with a serious illness have discovered the important role the spirit plays in our health and well-being. They've learned that when their spirit is strong and resilient, it can aid them in resisting even life-threatening diseases, and that a restful and bright spirit vastly improves their quality of life.

When it comes to experiencing all the energy we need, the condition of our spirit is extremely important. Here's why.

The Spiritual Potency in You

Our spirit is the part of us that, among other things, holds our highest values, our deepest dreams, and the "code" of rules by which we live. It's also the part of us that gauges how we're living in relation to what's important to us—not only to our values and dreams, but also to God, to other people, and to our sense of meaning or purpose. If we are in sync with these sources of personal vitality, our spirit is vibrant with the potent energies of love, peace, and happiness—real enthusiasm for living. But if we're out of sync in some significant way, our spirit is in tension. This deep-level angst drains us, not only of spiritual vitality, but of physical and mental energy as well.

The good news is, we can deal with deep-level tensions that drain us, and create new inner conditions that revitalize us at the core level of our being. Certain strategies can help give us more of the energy in spirit we need.

Spiritual Practices...for More Energy

Some of the strategies we'll be looking at in this chapter go by another name—*spiritual disciplines.*

This term comes from Christian spirituality. It refers to a set of practices that are known to strengthen and build our innermost being. Just as certain herbs are tonics for the body, you could say that spiritual disciplines are energizing tonics for the spirit. These techniques, some of them used for millennia, have the proven ability to create the kind of resilience and vitality that radiates throughout our whole being. They have been slightly updated here, and of course they're being applied to the business of creating more personal energy (though you may want to use them specifically to build healthier connections with yourself, with others, and with God).

If you want to release the deep-level conflicts that are draining you and rebuild a store of energy, try the following strategies to see which ones work for you.

THE SPIRITUAL ENERGY-BUILDING STRATEGIES

Strategy #1: Go on a Spiritual Quest

Spiritual boredom, or flatness, is a condition that leaves us low on energy. When we're bored in spirit, it's often because our relationship with God has gone flat. We're no longer on the inner quest to find our Source and understand ultimate truths.

Maybe you've had a longstanding relationship with God, but it's gone stale. Sure, God is out there..."but so what?" Or maybe you've decided that God is irrelevant or just too mysterious and elusive to bother with. But all faiths agree: God exists just out of reach of human abilities to comprehend...and human beings seem to be created to seek God.

There is an important bit of practical wisdom in this off-balance arrangement, though we often miss it. When things don't go our way we get cranky and want to sit down right where we are. We demand that God come around with a full explanation. We complain because we'd like to have God all figured out. (That way we'd know how to get God to do what we want all the time. But then we'd be God, wouldn't we?) Whoever set up this system had something else in mind—a dynamic arrangement that works in our favor.

"Seeking" is a state of being that gives us a spiritual energy that's like perpetual motion. The fact that God can be elusive and mysterious provides us with "fuel"—in the form of passionate *questions* that boost our "spiritual metabolism."

Do This:

Step 1: Set out to find God again. Make a list of the things you just don't "get" about God. "Who are you?" "How can I see you, hear you, know you?" "Where are you?"

Step 2: Let go of images of God that put you off. Some of us didn't have good parenting. Some may be distanced by the image of God as "a male." (For the record, the early Christian fathers and the Scriptures teach that God embodies both male and female.)

Step 3: Ask tough, honest questions. A spiritual quest is formed by the important questions we ask. Questions are catalytic. They rev us up and get us moving.

Many of us were raised to think that God is insulted or angered by our questions. Or we were told that some questions have no answer—implying that we should stop asking. If that's true for you, here's a suggestion: When you're approaching God, focus on the fact that many faiths—Christianity in particular—tell us God has a *welcoming* attitude. In a wonderful little scene from the Christian New Testament, Jesus showed us how we should come to God: "'*Let the little children come to me...*' *And he took the children in his arms...*"

When approaching God, be as *curious, open, honest...*and *boldly questioning...*as a little child.

Step 4: Remain alert and expect an answer to come…maybe when you least expect it. Here's the deeply re-energizing, final part of this strategy. Be open for an answer to come from *anywhere*. God is not limited and can "speak" to us anyplace, anytime…in every way possible.

When we begin the search for God and for deeper answers, we jump-start our spirit by triggering

→ focused interest

→ deep-level alertness

→ awakening to life's many dimensions

→ enthusiasm

Your Goal: With time you will begin to experience spiritually reawakened senses. Like the tingle you get when a limb has been "asleep," you will experience insights, realizations, wisdom—and also feel the energy that comes with the reawakening of *wonder* and *joy in discovery.*

Strategy #2: Create Sacred Space

Are you stressed? Too busy? Consumed by too much to do? Driven? Anxious?

This strategy, in a sense, counterbalances the previous one. Strategy #1 gets us moving again. Learning how to create sacred space trains us to slow down and experience deeply restorative spiritual rest. This strategy is similar to one in the previous chapter—but with a surprising twist added.

Do This:

Step 1: Make time to be alone and quiet. If your life is hectic this may take some effort. Find a place where you're not likely to be disturbed by other people. Be sure it's relatively free from noise and distractions.

Step 2: Re-collect your self. Busyness and stress scatter our focus. We feel pulled apart. We say things like "Boy, am I having a hard time keeping it all together." Our inner being is, as it were, being stretched thin. We re-collect ourselves by restoring restful focus. Here are some variations you can try:

~ **Focus on your breath…and its original Source.** Pay attention to the air as it moves in and out of your nostrils. Let your breathing relax, deepen, and slow. After a time, shift your focus to the sense of deep calm you experience…or…

Shift your focus to God…breathing life into all living things—including *you.*

~ **Focus on an image of God…from art or Scripture.** For some of us it's easier to focus attention on an image than on our breath. "Icons" are not that common in everyday life, but images of God are everywhere. After calming your breathing, shift your attention to an image from the world of great art…or one from the Bible.

~ **Focus on a Scripture. …** Then there are those of us who are stimulated by "hearing" more than "seeing." Try meditating on a favorite verse of Scripture—especially one that's positive and life-affirming. Repeat it slowly…almost like a chant.

~ **Open your imagination.** In a meditative state, some people have spiritual experiences that are visible only to the eye of the soul. These powerful connections with the divine are what sets this practice apart from the purely mental practice of clearing your head.

One workshop attendee "saw" herself gathering fragments of her stressed-out self back together and handing them to God, watching as God "reassembled" her. One man, listless and depressed at first, "saw" himself as empty…but then "watched" himself being slowly refilled with the energy of life again. After these experiences, both felt rested, refreshed, and re-energized.

Your Goal: You are learning how to re-connect with a sense of the divine and with God. Opening up a place in your busy life and in your inner being lets this re-connection take place. The more you practice this ancient spiritual discipline the more inner rest and available energy you will find.

Strategy #3: Spiritual "Housecleaning"

One of the great women of Christian spirituality, St. Teresa of Avila, described the human soul as an "interior castle." Okay, so it's hard these days to relate to the idea of living in a castle—but it can be useful to imagine your soul as a house with different rooms in it.

Some houses are bright and clean—"up" kinds of places. Others are dark and unpleasant, with a "down" feel to them. In the one we feel energetic; in the other we feel depressed or draggy.

Our spiritual house—that is, our soul—can harbor some unpleasant things that are definite energy-drainers. These are the darker attitudes and agitated moods. When these occupy our inner spaces, we will be lacking in positive energy—enthusiasm, buoyancy, spiritedness—that is generated from within and gives us vitality.

Maybe you wouldn't describe your soul as a dark or unpleasant "house"—but what about the closets and corners? Are there some "rooms" inside you where negative attitudes and moods collect... eventually spilling out? What's going on inside your spirit that wears you down?

Do This:

Step 1: Set aside time to be alone and quiet. With all that crams our schedules, it's hard to find time for personal reflection and the occasional look inward. If you're like most people, you'll have to *make* the time. Just be sure you go to a place where you're undisturbed. (And please—*turn off that cell phone!*)

Step 2: Conduct a thorough search. What are you looking for? Here are some of the attitudes to look for that may be draining you of vitality:

→ **Caustic attitudes**—superiority, judgmentalism, a cutting or catty spirit

→ **Soured attitudes**—cynicism, sarcasm, a petty and nit-picking spirit

→ **Dulling attitudes**—doubt, stubbornness, a "do it my way" spirit

→ **Deadening attitudes**—unwillingness to believe or trust, unforgiveness, hatred and anger, a despairing spirit

→ **Retreating attitudes**—fear, worry, laziness, complacency, a flat and uncaring spirit

Step 3: Visit the different "rooms" of your soul. Yes, you can push imagination too far, but if you need help with this essential self-examination—

→ **What's in the "attic"?** Are your *private thoughts* mostly negative or positive? Are your thoughts caught up almost 100-percent in the details of daily living, with little time set aside for personal escapes? Do you spend any time focusing on positive values and spiritual pursuits, like learning to be more patient, kind, generous, and loving, and being open to others' needs? Would your family, friends, and co-workers say you can be humble and open to others' directions—or are you most often unbending, insistent, needing to be in control, or bossy?

→ **What's in the living area?** Are your *relationships* comfortable, relaxed? Do your friends know they can count on you? Can you count on them? Or are your relationships strained? Do you feel mostly alone and isolated...or friendly and befriended?

→ **What's in the bedroom?** What about *intimate relationships?* Is there anyone with whom you can be totally open and vulnerable...and who still accepts you anyway? Or are you scared that if anyone really knew you—even your spouse or best friend—they'd be shocked, horrified, and disappointed?

→ **What's in the basement?** Are there unpleasant things from *your past*—things you've done, things others have done to you—stored in your soul? What is it that you've never really dealt with in a way that brings healthy resolution or rest?

Step 4: Choose just one area to work through. *Don't* try to get rid of everything at once. Doing what's called a "searching moral inventory" can be pretty overwhelming. (If you tend to be down on yourself, you also need to take an inventory of the good things you find in your spiritual house or you'll be ground to a pulp...and that's not the point of this strategy.) The point is to find harbored attitudes and life issues that are draining or hindering your spiritual vitality.

Step 5: Create a plan. Don't talk yourself out of it. When you know the one area that needs work, resolve to take action. Do you need a friend or confidant to share your burden with? Do you need to meet with someone from your past, or present, to resolve a major conflict or to make recompense?

If a nagging voice inside tells you, *Forget it—nothing will change,* that's the voice of hopeless despair. Don't let it weigh you down with chains and keep you spiritually stuck right where you are. Any time we make a step toward cleaning our spiritual house, we create more positive, spiritual energy. Depending on what you find you may want to

→ strengthen intimate and close relationships by honest, compassionate communication

→ seek help and counsel

→ ask forgiveness or make amends

Your Goal: Bad attitudes are those that keep us from engaging fully, freely, peacefully, and happily in life. Doing your part to empower a change gets your personal energy moving again—in the good direction.

Strategy #4: Let God Be the Care-Giver

Among the five billion people on this planet, some of us are Care-givers...with a capital C. Other people love to see us coming— our families, friends, bosses, co-workers, neighbors—because we invariably step in and start taking care…of people, problems, *anything* that needs to be taken care of.

While care-giving is a genuinely good spiritual trait in itself, how we use that trait can become harmful, not only to us but to other people as well. We can overperform and burn ourselves out while allowing other people to underperform and be lazy and never learn important living skills. Then we experience a deep-soul exhaustion…and come to resent or even hate the people we set out with such good intentions to love in our "caring" way. If this sounds tiringly familiar…

Do This:

Step 1: Make a list of all the people you do caring things for. Simple enough—right?

Step 2: Make a list of what you do for each person. A little more time-consuming…but there's a payoff coming!

Step 3: Honestly assess which of these things each person would be better off doing for themselves. This is the point where you will discover whether you are a *care-taker* or a *care-giver.* What's the difference?

Care-*givers* stand back and watch to see if other people need a hand—a bit of help doing what they have to do, or maybe some guidance on how to do it. Care-givers take on responsibilities *temporarily* and hand them back to their owners *quickly, cleanly,* and *happily.*

Care-*takers,* on the other hand, look for needs they can take on— even if other people are perfectly capable of doing these things by themselves. Sure, it's nice to lift someone else's burdens once in a while when they're sick or down or overwhelmed or otherwise unable to help themselves. But if we're care-takers rather than care-givers, we go too far. We need to be needed. Caring for others is how we get them to like us or love us back.

It is truly better for each one of us—including those beloved people we care-take—to learn how to be responsible for ourselves. Care-takers turn other people into dependents. Care-givers help other people know how to do things for themselves by passing on the skills of living. This makes the people they care about more sturdy, resilient, and self-confident.

So—which one are you? Care-*taker*…or care-*giver*?

Step 4: Give responsibilities back to the people they belong to. You may need to explain to people who are now overdependent on you that you can't handle the load any longer. They may not like it.

You may also need to do some training of those people. Write out directions or walk them through the steps. Let them know, "I'll run through this with you…and I'll be here if you have questions. But the responsibility for this task has to become yours."

Step 5: Entrust the other person's well-being to God. Mixed in with our need to be needed there is usually genuine care and concern for these other people. Unfortunately that "care" can become overconcern, worry, or fear. What if they don't pick up important responsibilities…and suffer for it?

Now it's time to trust that God will take care of these people as they learn how to care for themselves. Playing God—trying to keep these others from harm that's self-inflicted by their own irresponsibility—only wears us down…and it prevents them from becoming mature, healthy adults. Commit the other person to God's care. Remain in the picture, if you can, as a friend. Remind yourself, "God is their Source—I am only a *re*source."

Your Goal: When you transfer responsibilities back to their rightful owner…and commit this person to God's care…you recapture the energy drained from you by overwork and unnecessary worry.

Strategy #5: Try "Spiritual Weight Loss"

Lots of us carry around more weight than what's good for us—spiritual weight, that is.

Anxiety, depression, grief, unresolved hurt and anger, unpleasant secrets…these weigh our spirits down. They cause stress that drains energy, much the same way carrying a too-large physical load exhausts our bodies.

For centuries, people have relied on *spiritual confidants*—other people who can help us "shed" those energy-draining spiritual weights we carry. This is a person to whom you can bare your soul and off-load the inner weight that's sucking life energy out of you. This man or woman may be

→ a spiritual counselor

→ a confessor

→ a spiritual director

→ a spiritual friend

Do This:

Step 1: Find a member of the clergy, a paid counselor, or a wise friend with whom you can establish a "confessional relationship." Make it clear from the beginning that you are carrying some spiritual weights that are hard to shoulder alone and that you need help.

Step 2: Set up "ground rules." Make sure the following guidelines are clear:

~ **Whatever you talk about is confidential.** You need the freedom of safety so you can unburden your soul. The more we sense we're safe, the more we're able to disclose weighty matters.

~ **What you need first is encouragement.** You need support—not shame or belittlement, or someone to point out what you've done wrong.

~ **When you're ready for advice and the motivation to act, you'll ask for it.** And eventually you should. After establishing that your confidant supports *you* as a person...be ready to ask for advice, personal insight, and practical suggestions.

~ **Invite personal insights.** Sometimes we're in tough situations because of personal habits we can't see in ourselves. Sometimes we stay in tough situations because we're holding out for hopes, dreams, aspirations…but are doing so in the wrong setting or with the wrong person. Let your confidant know, "If you see something about me I don't see, feel free to talk about it."

~ **Actions and timing are up to you.** If you need to make changes in your life, *when* and *how* they get done has to be left up to you. After all, it's your life.

~ **If possible, create a long-term relationship.** Most human change comes about slowly. Wouldn't it be great if we could redirect our thinking, emotional connections and habits, and spiritual drives on a dime? Yes, it would—but it doesn't usually happen that fast.

Long-term confessional relationships are best. Why? Because most of us tend to return to old patterns of thinking and acting even when they have harmed us before. Longer relationships are not always possible, but when you can create them—by mutual agreement—they can help you not only to take the spiritual weight off…but keep it off.

Your Goal: We keep our spirits light by learning how to manage the matters that weigh us down. Keep yourself "fit" by spending time on a regular basis with a spiritual confidant.

Strategy #6: "Soul Stretching"

I once suggested to a workshop attendee that he might not be so chronically fatigued if he learned to forgive his father for past wrongs. "Oh right!" he snorted. "That would be a big stretch."

Exactly.

What's the first thing you do in the morning? *Stretch*—right? Stretching moves the lactic acid out of your muscles and allows newly oxygenated blood to flood in. This awakens and energizes your body.

There is a spiritual counterpart to stretching…and that is *offering forgiveness.*

Consider this: When we hold onto a wrong, we live with almost-constant subliminal tension. Our outlook on life can be gloomy, and our mood darker. Because we're not free and at ease, our muscles maintain a subtle tension and become rigid. It's like we're literally *carrying* offenses around with us. Because of this, unforgiveness becomes a major energy-drainer for many of us.

Forgiving *is* a spiritual "stretch"—because we have to reach further…maybe further than we've ever had to reach before…to extend grace to someone else.

Do This:

Step 1: Call to mind someone who has wronged you. You may have a list…but start with *one person*.

Step 2: Be clear in your thinking about exactly what they did wrong. "They lied about me" is too vague. "They lied about me and made me appear to be [dishonest, stupid, incompetent, a back-stabber]" is specific. *Be specific about the offense.*

Step 3: Be clear about the effects their wrongdoing had on your life. It isn't *just* the crime against us, hurtful as that was—the after-effects have been damaging, too.

Step 4: If possible, meet with the one who wronged you. A face-to-face meeting is important. You might want to take along a third party who can keep the conversation focused and forward-moving… not bogged down in the details of the offense, in blaming, or in arguing.

It may not be possible to meet with your offender…but there's another step to go.

Step 4: Stretch…by extending forgiveness. The other person obviously could not create the bonds of a good, healthy, life-affirming relationship. But maybe you can.

~ **Offer a chance to reconcile—a "goal" to shoot for.** "I'd like us to be friends again." "I'd like to have a good father–son/ father–daughter relationship." "Okay, we're strangers—but we don't have to be enemies."

~ **Engage in constructive dialogue.** Sure, you have to name the wrong that was done. But don't stay stuck there. "How can we make this right?" is the focus.

~ **Accept all offerings.** If someone can make a wrong right, graciously accept. Maybe even compliment them for doing the right thing. Sometimes the wrongs done to us are big and can't be made fully right again. (Not everything *can* be replaced this side of heaven.) All the offender may be able to offer are "tokens"—expressions of remorse, the promise of personal reform. These we graciously accept, too.

~ **"Release" the offender.** To release someone from a debt means conveying this message: "I will no longer hold this offense against you. You are not in my debt for anything."

~ **Rely upon God's grace.** God's grace is generally what makes forgiveness possible. In this case, grace gives us the right perspective—that is, the right way to see the whole situation.

   When we're wronged, our focus turns outward—onto the offender. We forget that we, as humans, have also wronged others whether we intended to or not. We have all done selfish, hurtful, or thoughtless things. But we don't like to see ourselves in this uncomfortable light, do we?

   Grace reminds us that we are imperfect—but that God's forgiveness is always extended to us. Grace puts us right next to the one who wronged us, right in the same boat! Just as we have needed forgiveness for our errors (and we're grateful when grace is extended to us!), others need forgiveness and are thankful for grace, too.

Your Goal: Let the life-giving, healing energy of forgiveness and grace move through you and out to those who wrong you. Then enjoy the revitalizing effect it has on your spirit.

Strategy #7: Get Passionate!

"The mass of men lead lives of quiet desperation," said one of our great philosophers—and so, of course, do many women. When

we have little or no passion for living, our inner jets burn very low...
and sometimes go out. Without passion, we become dull and
lethargic.

The good news is, your spark, your fire, your passionate spirit can
be reignited.

Do This:

**Step 1: Sort out your wants...and your desire to accomplish...
from your spiritual passion.** Many people mistake things on their
"want" list for their spiritual passion. Or they mistake their dream
of "accomplishing something great" for spiritual passion.

Spiritual passion arises out of a desire to enter into a situation
where there is hurt, loss, suffering, or need...and bring healing,
restoration, comfort, or blessing. A want connects us to a thing. A
desire to accomplish attaches us to a bigger, more shining mental
image of ourselves. A spiritual passion connects us to *other people.*

Ask yourself, "What hurt, loss, or suffering has touched me
deeply...personally? What need do I most want to fill?"

Step 2: Be wide open. Your passion may be to help kids who can't
read, or abused women, or elderly shut-ins. Or your passion may
be to lift people's spirits by creating beauty, or to keep things honest
by writing and reporting the truth. It may be to create a nurturing
home...or to give other people economic opportunities and good
services via a well-run business.

Step 3: Commit yourself to a time of transition. Maybe it's possible for you to stop doing what you're doing now...and step right
into the pursuit you're passionate about. For most of us, getting
there requires a time of transition. We need to take care of responsibilities...make plans...possibly get some training...find an oppor-
tunity.

Making a commitment to pursue your spiritual passion is crucial.
If we don't make commitments, it's too easy to give up and turn
back when the going is rough.

Consider making a commitment of your intent to

→   your parents or spouse

→   your clergyman, spiritual director, or friend

→   your church

Step 4: Lay out the "baby steps" that will get you there...and take the first one. As the well-known saying goes, "Every great journey begins with one step." Writing down the steps that will help you get to your spiritual passion gives you the "map." Taking the first small step gives you the joy and excitement of setting out on a new journey.

Your Goal: Reigniting the passion in your soul for living is very re-energizing. Some people think of it as a "new lease on life" or even a "spiritual rebirth." When you join the passion of your spirit with the pragmatics of a plan you too will experience a release of new spiritual energy.

In Closing

As crucial as it is to "fuel up" our inner being, we also need to pay careful attention to how we energize our body. In the next chapters, we'll turn to strategies for creating more physical energy.

5

The **More Energy** *Diet*

"I eat a *balanced diet*. I should have energy…right?"
"I eat lots of *protein*. I should have energy…right?"
"I eat lots of *carbohydrates*. I should have energy…right?"
"I eat almost *no fats*. I should have energy…right?"

Most of us have heard that certain types of food are "energy foods." We've also heard that we should cut down on other kinds of foods—especially fats. We're told we should eat a "balanced diet"— though we aren't told exactly what that means.

Then, of course, we've heard about food substances that give us bursts of energy…but then they wear off, leaving us fatigued again:

"When I feel tired, a chocolate bar picks me up for maybe an hour. But then I guess it wears off, and I suddenly feel wiped out."

"I drink caffeine just to get going in the morning. By mid-morning, when I'm fatigued again, I head for the coffeepot. I hit it again mid-afternoon, too. Or else I drink a cola. I probably drink a lot more caffeine than I should. But I should also have more energy than I do…right?"

The truth is, food substances like caffeine and refined white sugar *do* deliver an energy jolt. On the other hand, some medical experts tell us to avoid them altogether.

So often we're left with questions and confusion when it comes to this important aspect of living. For example, if eating "good food" and "balanced meals" is a chief source of energy, then why is it that even those of us who are more careful about what we eat *still* experience energy peaks and dips? We hear, "Eat more of *this*." "Drink less of *that*." What's the truth?

FUELING YOUR BODY: THE FUNDAMENTALS

The previous chapters offered strategies you can use to fine-tune your inner life and create reserves of mental and spiritual energy. Using the strategies presented in this chapter and the two that follow—on the work/rest cycle and natural supplements—will help you to experience even more physical vitality.

But first, when it comes to fueling your body, certain important "food-energy fundamentals" apply:

Food Fundamental #1: Eat "Mindfully"

Too many of us pay too little attention to what we eat. When we really pay attention we often make discoveries like the following:

→ **We eat too much...or too little.** Stress, hurry, boredom, fear of getting fat, fear of being skinny, overworking, underworking—lots of underlying factors cause us to eat more than we need, or less. The amount of fuel we're putting into our bodies doesn't match the amount we really need.

→ **We eat too much of one food type...and too little of another.** Often, the type of food we're eating doesn't match our energy needs. For instance, if we're working hard physically, but not eating enough complex carbohydrates to fuel us up, followed by enough proteins to rebuild stressed muscle tissues...we're actually breaking down muscle and exhausting ourselves. If we're more sedentary—say, working at a desk all day—we may be eating too many carbs and storing the energy as fat...again, making us sluggish.

→ **We graze in the "cheat zone" too often.** "Grazing" is actually a good way to eat, as we'll see in a moment. But *what we graze on* matters a lot. Generally speaking, the "little rewards" we indulge in fall into one of three categories:

• salty–crunchy

• sugary–chewy

• "mood lifters" (like caffeinated drinks) or "mood mellowers" (like alcoholic drinks)

Now, a *little* cheating is okay. The *occasional* sugar- or fat-laden dessert keeps us from feeling deprived. But grazing in the "cheat zone" too often ruins healthy energy production even if we're trying to eat right. (Imagine filling your car's gas tank with high-octane fuel…then sabotaging your own engine by dumping a fistful of mud in the tank.)

If we want more fuel from our food, we can have it by becoming more mindful about *what* we eat. This chapter will help you put together a menu of foods that are guaranteed to boost your energy levels.

Food Fundamental #2: Understand Your Natural Body Clock

Our body's real energy needs run on a natural cycle that we might depict like this:

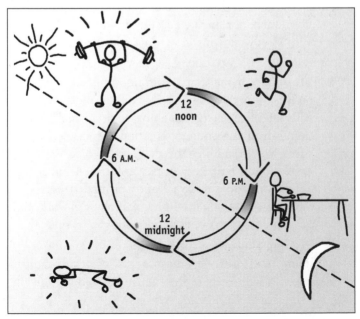

Here's what's going on throughout the course of an average person's daily cycle when he or she is in sync with the natural body clock:

→ **Midnight to dawn.** Throughout the night, our body's work is to "re-stock" the stores of biochemicals we'll need for the work of another day. If we learn how to cooperate with this cycle, we can wake up primed with the energy we need in order to start the day bright-eyed and with a spring in our step.

But if we make critical mistakes at bedtime—which most of us do—we'll counteract what our bodies need for energizing…maybe sleep poorly, too…and wake up groggy.

→ **Morning prime time.** From 6 A.M. or so through 12 noon, our body's energizing chemistry is at peak flow. With a little of the right reinforcement from energizing foods, we can boost our energy and extend "prime time" till well into the afternoon.

On the other hand, the common mistakes most of us make can deplete our energy rapidly. Sometime shortly after lunch, our mental and physical energy dips. We're a little sleepy, slowing down at work…and wishing the workday were over.

→ **Afternoon prime time.** From noon till about 6 P.M., our body is being called upon to put out the most effort. Along with supplying energy for a myriad of normal body functions—from digestion to repairing damaged cells and tissues—we are adding the day's workload. With a little know-how, we can keep ourselves fortified and energetic.

However, add emotional and spiritual stressors—and who doesn't have them?—on top of physical work, and we can rapidly overtax our energy resources by midday.

→ **Evening slowdown time.** In the early- to mid-evening hours, our stores of energy-producing hormones dip even lower. A light meal of the right foods can keep us on an even keel, with enough energy for an evening of enjoyable activity.

Many of us, however, opt for an evening meal dense in calories, which our body must work harder to digest—taxing our metabolism and further draining our energy. We wind up on a sofa for hours before bedtime...with food energy being stored as fat, which will weigh us down and tire us even more as the days go by.

→ **Back to...a night of restorative rest.** As our body clock winds down and we sink into sleep, we need to prime our body for the eight hours of restorative work it needs to do. How else will we be able to replenish those stores of energy-producing hormones? The right kind of bedtime snack will give our body the energy it needs to do its night-time work and will get us ready to wake "primed" with energy in the morning.

Unfortunately, too many of us eat snacks late in the evening that are laden with useless calories. Or we go to bed on an empty stomach, forcing our bodies to draw on energy stored in lean body tissues...so we wake feeling tired, or even drained.

How can we turn around the cycle of energy depletion that many of us experience?

Food Fundamental #3:
Graze on "Energy Foods"

As a culture, we've trained ourselves to eat three times a day—breakfast, lunch, and dinner (along with midday and bedtime snacking—usually from the "cheat zone"—which we usually don't count).

Generally speaking, our body chemistry has been designed so that we benefit more from eating in a "light grazing" pattern. This is because we need a source of energy to produce energy—and we need it in a more constant supply than eating "three square meals a day" gives us. Our energy level will remain more constant if we

→   eat the right combination of energy-producing foods

→   eat more frequently—as many as three smaller meals and three healthy snacks each day

Given what we know about the body's 24-hour energy needs, a better eating pattern looks like this:

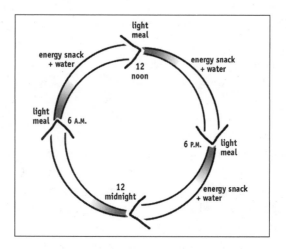

In the "More Energy Diet" that follows, we'll discuss the best energy-producing foods. We'll also talk about the best combination in which to eat them in order to release their vitalizing nutrients.

WHY YOU NEED TO
DRINK MORE WATER

∼

It can be confusing.

You want to take natural supplements…and the advice is, *Give them time to work because their therapeutic potency builds up gradually in your system.*

At the same time you're told, *Be sure to drink more water.*

But doesn't water *dilute* substances and make them weaker?

The fact is, you do need to drink more water when taking natural supplements (and, for that matter, prescription drugs, too). Water does *not* dilute the potency of natural supplements, and it *does* help flush the kidneys and liver. This is very important because these two vital organs may already be taxed when we're feeling tired or exhausted. Flushing them by drinking more water will relieve stress and help them function at peak capacity.

Start by drinking four 8-ounce glasses of water a day. Over a period of one to two weeks, increase your intake to eight 8-ounce glasses a day. This may sound like a lot of water, but your body will adjust.

In fact, since mild dehydration is also a common cause of fatigue, you may find that drinking more water gives your energy levels a great natural boost.

Remember to drink cool water—not ice-cold water, which causes your body to experience the symptoms of mild shock—*especially* on hot days.

Food Fundamental #4: A"30-40-30" Balance Means Energy

So far, we're becoming 1) more aware of what we actually eat, 2) aware that our body's natural rhythm requires energy at points in the day that differ from our normal eating schedule, and 3) aware that we need to eat smaller, more energizing meals throughout the day to give our body what it really needs to steadily produce energy.

The fourth important food fundamental is this: If we want the most available energy from our foods, we need to eat in the right balance—which means, in terms of calories, eating *30 percent protein, 40 percent carbohydrates, and 30 percent fat at any given meal or snack.*

Of course, this means eating the most beneficial proteins, carbs, and fats, and we'll look at what those are in a moment. For now, it's important to understand the 30-40-30 combination and why it delivers the energy we need.

Research shows that eating in this 30-40-30 balance naturally stimulates our metabolism. It does this by triggering the production of hormones in a combination that feeds every system of our body what it needs for healthy, efficient functioning. And it does so in a way that also helps our body use stored fat as well. So, energy-wise, eating a 30-40-30 balance gives us a fantastic supply of ready vitality…*without* adding fat to our body.

"Now hold on," you may be saying. "I can understand why getting 30 percent of my calories from protein and 40 percent from carbs is a healthy way to eat. But getting *30 percent of my calories from fat?* That sounds like a *lot of fat.*"

Actually, it's not. Fat is far more calorie-dense than either protein or carbohydrates. In fact, it takes a *very small amount* of fat to give you 30 percent of the total calories per meal you need.

So let's say you're putting together a 30-40-30 breakfast, beginning with oatmeal and skim milk as your basis.

Do this:

Step 1: Count the protein calories in the oats and milk to come up with your "30-percent protein" number. Let's say it's *90 calories from protein*. (This means you'll be aiming for about 300 calories total to fill out your meal. You may have to do some converting from grams.)

Step 2: Now you'll need about *120 calories from carbohydrates* to reach your "40-percent carbs" goal. You count the carb calories in the oats and milk and find they total, say, 80. You'll need to add 40 more calories from carbs—which you can easily do by adding some of your favorite fresh fruit.

Remember this: Sugar is not a beneficial carbohydrate. It may give you a quick shot of energy, but you'll burn it off fast...and then comes the energy crash. You're better off learning to enjoy the taste of fruit as your natural sweetener.

Step 3: Now you need 30 percent of your meal to come from fat calories. This means you need about *90 calories from fat* to reach your 300-calorie total. Again, fatty foods are much more calorie-dense than either proteins or carbs...so you'll only need a very small amount of fat to give you your 90 calories. You might add 1 small pat of butter... *or* 2 or 3 slivered almonds...*or* stir in 1 teaspoonful of peanut, almond, or cashew butter. *That's all the fat you need.*

Believe it or not, it only takes a little practice to learn how to create meals in this balanced, 30-40-30 combination. And the benefit—more energy—will far outweigh the little bit of conscious effort it takes to read the nutrition labels on food packages and to do the minor amount of math required to rebalance your favorite meals and snacks...turning them into energizing events.

Now that you've got these basics, it's important to know what kind of diet can deliver all the nutritional energy you need. Because tastes and preferences are so individual, it will be up to you to assemble lists—from the proteins, carbs, and fats recommended below—that will work into a satisfying diet for you.

THE "MORE ENERGY DIET"

What kind of diet delivers all the energy we need? The answer is...

1. A diet that combines

→ **vital proteins**—those that release the most amino acids for creating strength and endurance...and demand the least amount of energy for digestion

→ **vital carbohydrates**—those that fuel the body for quick energy...instead of triggering the body's "fat-storage" response

→ **vital fats**—those that are necessary for every major bodily function...and are least likely to become toxic, or be stored exactly where you don't want it, or both

2. Eating these vital nutrients in the *right, 30-40-30 balance* for the *majority* of your meals and snacks.

Diets and eating plans abound these days. Most are focused on weight loss. Unfortunately, many of these diets—even some of the most popular—have been created as if losing weight is the only important goal we can have. Weight loss or weight management is important. But equally important goals are

→ **giving our bodies enough energy to perform every important function**—from metabolism, to work and family demands, to recreational pursuits, to replenishing necessary stores of biochemicals

→ **eating the kinds of foods that increase our metabolism**—giving us all the energy we need...*while* allowing our weight to settle itself at a healthy level

Proteins...to Increase Your Strength

The foundation of a great "More Energy Diet" is proteins—the right kind of proteins.

EAT FOR ENERGY...
AND THE POUNDS WILL GO, TOO

〜

Unfortunately, many of today's most popular diets *do not* support our body's needs when it comes to energy production...or even good health. So while you may lose weight, you can also find yourself getting fatigued.

Worse, many dieters set in motion an unhealthy cycle—beginning with hormonal depletion and resulting in the suppression of their immune system.

Sadly, as the vast majority of dieters also discover, once they go off a diet that's aimed only at weight loss, their bodies "boomerang." They gain back all those pounds they fought to take off and—because they've depressed their metabolism—they may gain even *more* weight. Many find this to be the case even if they've changed their lifestyle and become more active. This is not only ironic, it's both sad and unnecessary.

Bottom line: When you eat for your body's real energy needs you are far more likely to lose weight (if that's your need) and keep it off...*or* maintain a healthy weight—that is, the weight that's appropriate for the activities you need to accomplish in your day.

Most important, you'll be focused on good health, which increases longevity and the real enjoyment of life...long after you stop looking good in a leotard or bathing suit.

Certain types of proteins promote overall vitality because they're high in amino acids, but they don't take a lot of energy to digest *and* they create minimal toxicity as they break down. Other proteins stress our bodies. They require more energy to digest, tax our hormonal output, and leave destructive toxins circulating through our bodies.

If you want to eat for energy, what are your best protein choices?

#1 Protein Choice: Plant Proteins

Most of us find it hard to believe that plants can deliver enough protein to make us strong and energetic. With our ingrained stereotypes, we just can't picture a lumberjack, a construction worker, or a cattle rancher sitting down to a hefty soy burger at the end of a hard day's work. If you're going to build healthy muscle tissue and have strength, you need meat—right? (Wrong.)

Many plant proteins contain the same amino-acid profile as meat. They don't tax the body's hormonal system, because they're easier to digest than meats, making their energy more readily available to tissues and cells. As they break down they create fewer toxins to be eliminated from the body.

And here's a very important factor: Plant proteins are far lower in damaging fats than animal proteins. Whereas animal fats tend to be higher in the omega-6 fatty acids—the kind that boost your LDL, or "bad" cholesterol—the right kinds of plant proteins contain a balance of omega-3 and omega-6 fatty acids. So they keep your HDL and LDL cholesterols more balanced…just what the doctor ordered.

If you're concerned about cancer—maybe because you've had a personal scare or because it runs in your family—here's a final piece of good news about plant proteins. Many doctors recommend a diet high in plant protein and low in (or without) animal proteins. That's because tumors can "feed" on the omega-6 fatty acids contained in meats. And further, there's a greater level of toxicity created by meat digestion, which depletes your body of energy as it works hard to eliminate the toxins. All of these factors bring doctors to the conclusion that meat consumption generally works counter to your immune system…which adds up to the fact that plant protein is a far better choice, *especially* for those of us for whom cancer is a concern.

So what plant proteins make the most energy available to us? Though the grains here are often listed among the carbohydrates (brown rice, for instance, is an almost perfect carb) they're listed here also (whereas other grains are not) because of their higher protein content.

Here are your top choices:

- **Barley** is as high in protein as meat. People in many cultures actually work hard and thrive on a diet based on barley. As for its uses in cooking, barley is a highly versatile grain that can be eaten as a cooked cereal, mixed into soup, or baked into bread.

- **Brown rice.** Two factors make this grain a great source of energy. First, it's rich in the B vitamins, which are needed to support every major system of your body. Second, it falls in the middle of the glycemic index, which means that it doesn't make your blood-sugar levels spike and drop.

- **Oats.** Today, oats are being promoted as a "heart-healthy" choice—and they are. But a simple bowl of oatmeal, as a meal or snack, provides a great balance of proteins *and* carbohydrates…delivering readily available energy.

- **Quinoa** (*"keen-*wah") has the highest protein of any grain—16 percent—*and* it's a complete protein, which means it has an amino-acid profile much like milk. It's rich in natural iron, in the B vitamins, and in vitamin E. Quinoa is easy to digest, making its energy quickly available to the body.

- **Soy** is yet another excellent source of plant protein. To make things easier, there is a wide range of soy food on the market today—like soy milk, soy cheese, soy burgers, soy mayonnaise, soy sausage, soy bacon, and soy yogurt. (If your first experiences with soy foods were not good—and mine weren't—you'll be happy to know that the makers of soy products have been working hard to make them taste good, too.)

#2 Protein Choice: Fish

Fish is an excellent source of lean protein (ever seen a fat fish?). And fish oil contains a range of omega-3 and omega-6 fatty acids—supplying your body with the full range of essential fatty acids (EFAs) it needs, along with protein.

What follows is a list of recommended fish and other seafoods, with those containing the most EFAs on top:

✴ anchovies, herring, mackerel, salmon

✴ albacore tuna, sablefish, sardines

✴ bluefin tuna, trout

✴ halibut, swordfish

✴ freshwater bass, oysters

✴ sea bass

✴ pollock, shrimp

✴ catfish, crabs

✴ clams, cod, flounder, scallops

#3 Protein Choice: Poultry

Poultry, the so-called "white meat," can be a good source of protein energy. *But it depends on the supplier and on how you prepare your poultry.*

Some poultry raisers "feed out" their animals in a way that "fattens" them for market. This means you're getting meat loaded with unhealthful fats. So what can you do to be a wise consumer of poultry products?

→ **Read the labels.** Those of us who are conscientious about our health have switched to eating free-range chickens raised on grain containing DHA. This keeps them leaner, and it makes their meat high in both the omega-3 and omega-6 EFAs. You'll find this information on the label.

→ **Eat baked or broiled, not fried.** Battering or frying chicken or turkey *does* make the meat flavorful. But it also loads the meat with fat, wiping out the healthful benefits. Baking or broiling in a manner that allows the fats to drip off is the healthiest way to cook poultry.

So onto your menu go…

• chicken (free-range/DHA-fed)

- turkey (free-range/DHA-fed)

- eggs (from free-range/DHA-fed poultry)

#4 Protein Choice: Red Meats

We've already gone through a list of red meat's energy-draining effects on the body. Is there any place for red meats in a healthy diet? Are there any that give our bodies more energy than is required for digestion?

Here are some tips:

→ **Eat red meats sparingly.** Dr. Barry Sears, developer of the widely successful Zone Diet, suggests we use red meat "like a garnish." Top your barley, brown rice, or quinoa with a small amount of red meat and you can still enjoy the flavor while giving your body a healthy dose of energizing protein.

→ **Eat the leanest cuts.** Ask your butcher to point out the very leanest cuts of red meat. Some grocers label red-meat products, and you can often find prepacked red meats that contain minimal fat—as low as 7 percent.

→ **Broil or bake red meat.** As with all meats, you want to allow as much grease as possible to drip free so that you're not putting extra animal fats, and the toxins they create, into your body.

Your Protein-Energy Goal: To turn any meal or snack into an energy-producing event, make it your goal to get about 30 percent of your calories from the top-choice proteins.

Carbohydrates...for Quick and Lasting Energy

As with proteins, certain carbohydrates are better sources of energy than others.

Simple Carbohydrates

Simple carbohydrates are higher on the glycemic index. This means they turn to sugar quickly, and that triggers rapid insulin production. How does this affect you? It gives you quick energy…but the "rush" fades quickly, sometimes in just a few minutes. You may even experience an energy crash. (That's why, for instance, the load of simple carbs you get from eating a chocolate bar can "pick you up"…but then a half-hour later you may suddenly need a nap.)

Complex Carbohydrates

Complex carbohydrates are lower on the glycemic index. Their energy is released a little more slowly than that of simple carbs—but its effects are much longer lasting. All told, complex carbs are a much better choice if you need quick *and* lasting energy.

So, what complex carbs should you eat to have the sustained energy you need?

Fruits. Fruits contain *fructose,* a form of sugar that releases its energy slowly during digestion. They are also rich in other phytochemicals your body needs for energy boosting. Some fruits contain natural substances that are as energy-boosting as caffeine— apples, for instance, are rich in *quercetin.* For sustained energy, keep on hand

- apples
- bananas
- blueberries
  (fresh or frozen)
- grapes
- mangoes
- papayas
- pears
- pineapple
- strawberries (fresh or frozen)
- raisins (1/3 cup of dried fruit is
  plenty)
- raspberries (pricey, but good for
  a treat)

Oranges, grapefruits, tangerines and other citrus fruits deliver ready, natural energy—but their acidity can become a problem.

Vegetables. Mom said, "Eat your veggies. They're good for you." But not all vegetables are the same. Some are high in starches, and they increase insulin production…triggering fat storage. Go lightly on vegetables like *corn, green peas, potatoes, sweet potatoes, yams,* and *yuccas (cassavas).*

Better energy-producing choices are

- **cruciferous vegetables**—bok choy, broccoli, cabbage, cauliflower, kohlrabi
- **dark-green leafy vegetables**—alaria (wakame), arame, dulse, hijiki, kombu, nori, sea palm (all of these are sea plants)
- **legumes**—adzuki, garbanzo beans (chickpeas), great northern beans, lima beans, navy beans
- **light-green leafy vegetables**—kale, red-leaf lettuce, romaine, spinach

Grains. We've already discussed the top-choice energizing grains in the "proteins" section earlier. You may have noticed that *wheat* was not listed. Despite the prevalence of bleached(-out) wheat flour in the Western diet, much better grain choices to improve your intake of energizing complex carbs are these:

• amaranth	• oat
• barley	• rye
• quinoa	• soy
• kamut	• spelt
• millet	• stone-ground whole wheat

Most of these grains can be purchased ground as flour. With a little practice, they make excellent substitutes for white flour in baking and cooking. Others make delicious and glycemically balanced cooked cereals. When mixed with fresh fruit, they'll give you great breakfast or snack-time energy.

Your Carbohydrate-Energy Goal: First you made a great protein choice. Now add to your meal or snack some of the top-choice carbohydrates listed here—so they make up about 40 percent of the calories in what you're about to eat.

Fats...for Long-Haul Energy

If you're expecting to hear that certain fats are more healthful for you than others *and* that they're also better sources of energy...you're right.

Some fats do not metabolize well. During digestion, they contribute little to healthy body functions, they're likely to become toxic in your system or elevate your cholesterol level or both...and if that's not bad enough, what's not eliminated will be stored as body fat.

On the other hand, *some* fat in your diet is absolutely necessary to keep your body functioning in a healthy, energetic way. It's very important not to eliminate all fat from your diet, not even for weight-loss purposes. In fact, *eating the right amount of fat, in combination with protein and carbohydrates, boosts your metabolism and helps you lose unhealthy body fat.* It's also very important to eat the right kinds of fat—those that contribute to healthy body function— if you want to have energy resources to draw on throughout the day.

→ **Eliminate or greatly reduce these fats.** We've already discussed the need to greatly limit your intake of animal fats. Other fats you should try to eliminate or reduce in your diet include *canola oil (in cooking—cold use is fine), coconut oil, palm oil, and peanut oil.*

→ **Use these fats—sparingly.** Fats that are more healthful, and also beneficial in boosting energy—when used *lightly*—include the following.

Butters:

- almond butter
- cashew butter
- cow's-milk butter
- olive oil–butter spread

Oils:

- fish oil
- flax oil
- hemp oil
- olive oil
- sesame oil

Seeds and nuts:

- almonds
- pumpkin seeds
- cashews
- sesame seeds
- peanuts

Your Fat-Energy Goal: You've got a plate that's holding 30 percent top-choice protein calories…and 40 percent top-choice carbohydrate calories. Now if you get 30 percent of your calories from top-choice fats—*you've put together an energizing meal or snack!*

Remember: As you saw in "Food Fundamental #4, it takes a very small amount of fat to give you all you need to turn a meal or snack into an energizing event.

In Closing

Retraining yourself to eat in a 30-40-30 balance *will* give you more energy. Adapting to a "grazing" pattern will spread your energy intake throughout the day and support your body through its cycle of real energy needs. You'll wish you'd known this long before now!

However, as important as balanced and timed eating are to giving us energy…there is another major factor to address. The fact is, our bodies need to have an *"energy demand"* put on them—a workload—to help them function at-peak. Too much of a physical demand, and we drain ourselves. Not enough, and we don't get our metabolism "up and running" enough to experience a satisfying energy flow. In short, we are made in such a way that we have to expend the right amount of energy to feel and enjoy that energy.

In the next chapter, we'll consider how to put the right kind of demand on our bodies—especially in terms of healthy exercise—to experience the energy flow we need for good health and well-being.

6

The Work/Rest Cycle

I'm working a full-time job *and* going to school full-time. How can I have all the energy I need so I can do everything that's got to be done?"

"I'm a single mom, working and raising three kids. I try to devote time to my church. I'd also like to have some kind of life of my own. 'Like to' is the operative term. If I just had more energy…"

"My boss is pushing me to work 16-hour days. If I just hold on and keep hammering away for the next few years, I'll make the career breakthrough I need. How can I have enough energy to keep from getting all these colds and illnesses I'm picking up? And to keep my relationships from suffering?"

"I get a good night's sleep. But I never seem to wake up during the day. All day long I'm dragging."

"I wish I were young again. I could get up and go, go, go through the whole day…and still have energy left to go out and have fun at night."

Does This Sound Like You?

Most of us wish we could find that "fountain of youth" again. Or at least we want the *energy* of youth…minus the foul-ups and missed opportunities of our younger days. (Welcome to the human race.)

By now, you may have realized that having enough energy—all that we need to get through our day—requires us to maintain a set of balances that deliver that energy when we need it. Yes, it would be great if we *could* tap into some amazing source of energy and feel it flow perpetually…like that fountain of youth we wish for. What's really needed, though, is a slightly more realistic approach to ourselves and our energy needs.

WORKING WITH YOUR BODY: THE FUNDAMENTALS OF PHYSICAL ENERGY FLOW

In the last chapter, we explored four fundamental principles for getting enough energy from the food we eat. What we need, to complete the picture, are some basic principles about our bodies' work/rest cycle. Call these the fundamentals of *body energy*.

Body-Energy Fundamental #1: Understand Your Body's Natural Energy Cycle

Each of us has a natural energy cycle. There are many variations, of course. To get a basic understanding, consider two common scenarios.

Running on Adrenaline

Let's say you're a "morning person," one of those people who can, more or less, plunge into your day with lots of energy. Your tendency may be to launch into your day "firing on 18 cylinders." You are a ball of energy. Even though you feel yourself starting to sag a bit by lunchtime, your momentum keeps you moving, running on adrenaline, till mid- or late afternoon. The problem is, when you're spent...you're *really* spent. Stick a fork in you, because your ability to be energetic is *done*.

While it's "natural" for some of us to be "up," and to go, go, go until we're "running on adrenaline," few of us recognize when that pattern begins to change...and even work against us. Over a long period of time—years—your up-and-running time gets shorter and shorter. Pretty soon, you can cook like a barn on fire until, maybe, only noon. Then...you're good until only late morning...*maybe*.

There is a parallel problem that can also occur—and it's important enough to stop and consider it, too. As your peak-energy time is dropping, you may also begin to experience more illness and injury. Perhaps you even develop a chronic illness…or a chronic condition you had in childhood suddenly gets much worse.

At this point, many of us find some outside force to pin the blame on: aging; "those people and all their demands"; "life"; bad "luck of the draw" when they fished you out of the gene pool.

The truth is, many of us who are like this run out of energy because we are experiencing *adrenal depletion.*

Adrenal depletion, besides leaving us wiped out, is actually a very real and serious health problem. The adrenal glands, which sit atop the kidneys, regulate not only energy supply, but also supply energy to your body's immune system. When you've expended the energy from the food that's racing around in your bloodstream, then dipped way into the glycogen stores in your muscles, you finally come to a point where you are "running on adrenaline." Run down your adrenaline stores, and over time you burn up one of the *main sources of energy for your immune system.* Immune suppression can lie at the root of many devastating illnesses and chronic health conditions. When we've stressed our adrenals, care is needed—beginning with right nutrition, and also with getting ourselves into the right work/rest cycle. With time—and hopefully with new wisdom about our real limits—adrenal depletion can be reversed.

Of course you may not trigger immune suppression to such a devastating degree. But you may, nonetheless, be in the daily habit of dipping into your adrenaline supplies. Some medical experts say we can even become, in a sense, addicted to our own adrenaline the way some people are hooked on, say, caffeine.

Okay, so you may not blast off like a rocket each morning…but your best energy does come earlier in the day. How can you have *more* energy *throughout* the day? Before we answer that question, consider this second scenario.

Never Quite in Gear

Then again, some of us feel like we never do get energized. We wake up slowly…and continue to feel like we're in "wake-up mode" for most of the day. Maybe we actually do feel awake at *some* point in the day. But energetic? That's another matter. Unfortunately, the real world requires us to be up and functioning, working on *its* time schedule, not ours, and kicking in some energy to get things done.

Oddly enough, many of us who are like this find that our energy can suddenly peak at odd hours of the day. At work, when we need energy, it's as if we're sleepwalking…but then we feel energized on the commute home. Or we can hardly keep our eyes open at the supper table, when the family needs our attention…but then we're up late, channel surfing, when we need to be asleep.

The truth is, we may already have all the energy we need—but we're not doing enough to trigger the biochemical reaction that we would experience as energy. Picture a stack of dry wood with enough good kindling under it…but no match to strike to get the fire crackling.

Those of us who feel lethargic (when mentally or spiritually based depression is not the cause) may in fact be experiencing a physiological kind of "depression" when we "just can't get going."

Pushing through the low parts of your cycle *without caring for yourself with nourishment and rest* may seem like the adult thing to do. But it's a formula for adrenal depletion, exhaustion, and possibly even illness. On the other hand, *caring for yourself can mean working enough to get your body's natural energy cycle started.*

What *is* your body's natural energy cycle? When are you most alert and energetic? When are you slowing down?

Body-Energy Fundamental #2: You Need to Expend Energy to Create Energy

In the two scenarios we just laid out, one type of person expends physical energy—but they do it virtually all at once, something like a rocket's booster engines. After the blast, after burning off all the fuel, these people experience a sudden drop-off in energy. The other type of person seldom feels those boosters ignite, so everything from takeoff to landing is a very slow flight.

Both types, oddly enough, can benefit by learning the same fundamental principle of energy creation: You have to expend energy to create energy—that is, the right energy.

To expend the "right energy" means two things: First, it means *expending enough physical energy to boost our metabolism to "work pace."* Second, it means *learning to keep the energy flow going as long as it's needed by working at a steady pace.*

In the last chapter, we learned how to put the right kind of "fuel in our tanks." In this chapter we'll now learn strategies that "turn the key and put the vehicle in gear"…and keep it running at a good pace throughout most of the day.

Body-Energy Fundamental #3: You Need Enough Rest to Create Energy

The other absolute essential needed to create physical energy is *rest*.

Medical research tells us that most of us adults are sleep-deprived. Sleep deprivation not only robs us of energy, it depresses every aspect of our being—mental, spiritual, and physical. All the functions of the body suffer, including immunity and metabolism.

A sluggish person can exist in a sleep-deprived state just as much as an "energetic" one. On the one hand, we can push ourselves too hard, training ourselves to get by on less sleep and rest. On the other hand, we can be too easy on ourselves, walking around feeling sluggish and half-dozy all day…and then drop into bed for a night of restless sleep. In both cases, we can wake fatigued because we're not getting enough of the deep sleep we need to really replenish our stores of energy.

Sleep and rest give our bodies a chance to replenish the stores of biochemicals that generate energy. (As mentioned in the previous chapter, a little of the right foods before bedtime can keep our metabolism running at a low level that doesn't deplete our energy—but helps add to it by continuing to circulate nutrients for cell growth and repair while we sleep.) For this reason, we need strategies that will give us essential rest—not just at night, but even at natural low points during our body's daily natural energy cycle. (Waiting till the weekend, or till an upcoming vacation, to catch up on sleep is not one of them.)

Obviously, there are individual needs—such as state of health, menstruation, and workload—that you'll have to factor in. But what follows are strategies to help you *replenish energy*—some of which you can use anytime, anywhere—and *increase your endurance* so you can feel energetic over a longer period of time.

Bottom line: Learning how to both *work* and *rest* in a way that's more in sync with the energy demands of your daily schedule is one of the greatest things you can do to care for yourself.

THE ENERGY-REPLENISHING STRATEGIES (REST)

These simple strategies will help you experience energy-replenishing rest during times of your day when you feel fatigued but have "more day to go." They will also help you experience more deeply-restorative sleep if you use them before bedtime or a nap.

Strategy #1: Stretch to Release "Stored Stress"

Throughout the day we all experience various forms of stress—mental, spiritual, emotional, and physical. Unfortunately, even non-physical stresses translate into physical tension, and stress can wind up being stored in our muscles. We experience tension headaches, stiff muscles, sore backs, painful muscle knots, pinched nerves...and then feel groggy. All because of stored tension.

This body-based kind of fatigue comes from a buildup of lactic acid in our muscle tissues. Our muscles have literally tensed—either to resist an "impact," or in preparation to do more work. In this "tensed for fight or flight" state, they're resisting the flow of oxygenated blood and retaining the lactic acid that builds up when they work. It's this lack of oxygenation that we experience as fatigue and weakness…and this buildup of lactic acid that we experience as stiffness and pain.

And so we feel tired from our exertion and need rest—but what happens? We feel fatigued, but we're unable to settle into a night's sleep or a nap…or even just kick back and relax. The tension stored in our bodies actually prevents us from getting the sleep or rest we crave.

Here's a simple strategy you can use anytime or anywhere you find yourself in the grip of tension. It's especially effective just before turning in at night, as well as when you're in need of a restorative nap.

Do This:

Step 1: Take a comfortable position, either sitting or lying down. Never force a stiff muscle. All your movements should be slow and gentle. The goal is to press lactic acid out of your muscles and trigger a relaxed state. Repeat each step that follows until the muscle group being worked relaxes. *Remember to breathe slowly and deeply while you stretch.*

Step 2: Release the tension in your neck. Just holding up an eight-and-a-half-pound head all day is a lot of work for those neck muscles. Then there's all the work your facial muscles do—talking, chewing, smiling, frowning. Plus the tension we store in our neck when stress hits. That's a lot of tension stored in those narrow, sinewy muscles.

Never roll your head to stretch tense neck muscles, as this can damage the delicate vertebrae in your neck. Instead,

→   Begin by turning your head to the right. Then drop your chin until it touches your collarbone. Then go back to the resting position.

→   Now repeat on the left side.

Continue to stretch…and release…until you've relieved the tension in the group of muscles that runs from each shoulder blade up the back of your neck. Continue this pattern through the following steps.

Step 3: Release your upper back.

→ Raise your left shoulder toward your ear. At the same time, push your shoulder forward, and feel the muscles between your spine and shoulder blade stretch. Return to resting position.

→ Do the same thing for your right shoulder.

Step 4: Release your chest and abdominals.

→ Extend your arms in front, palms down, and lay one hand on the other.

→ Slowly raise your straightened arms up over your head, inhaling and allowing your diaphragm to expand.

→ Reach for the sky, allowing your chest and abdominal muscles to stretch. Relax…but keep your arms raised.

→ Now clasp your hands together. Use your left arm to draw your right arm across your face. Feel the muscles down the back of your right ribs stretch.

→ Repeat for the benefit of your left side.

Step 5: Release your upper leg muscles (standing or seated).

→ With your arms outstretched, hands one over the other, slowly bend at the waist and reach for your left foot. Keep your left leg as straight as possible. Feel the buttock and hamstring muscles stretch. Return to the relaxed position.

→ Repeat for the right side.

Step 6: The "rolling" stretch (standing or lying down). This stretch should be done like a wave—gathering energy and momentum, slowly moving up your body more and more, until you're totally stretching.

→ Point your toes…relax…point your toes *and* flex your calf muscles…relax…

→ Point toes, flex calves…flex your quadriceps (upper leg muscles)…relax

→ Repeat—each time beginning with your toes and moving up your body

…next time pinching your buttocks

…then stretching your torso by opening your diaphragm

…finally, extending your arms and reaching as far as you can

When you finish with this full-body stretch you will have stimulated the movement of lactic acid out of your muscles and into the bloodstream for elimination. And you'll feel relaxed and tranquil…ready for refreshing, restorative sleep.

PILATES AND YOGA

While we're on the subject of a good energizing stretch… Pilates ("pih-*lah*-teez"—named after the developer of the method, Joseph Pilates) and yoga are excellent personal practices that will give you more energy. There are some similarities in these two practices—mainly, that they increase flexibility and strength while gently boosting your metabolism.

You can find Pilates classes and yoga classes through your local health club or community center. Yoga, though it is sometimes taught as an Eastern meditation practice, is also taught by many instructors minus the spiritual philosophies…so opt for that if you're not interested in the metaphysics.

Best of all, once you know the routines and moves, you can use them yourself any time of the day you feel cramped, restless, or tense. They will increase blood and oxygen flow and leave you feeling lightly buoyant, with restored vitality.

Strategy #2: "Walk to Sleep"
or "Walk to Wake"

Walking can deliver a nice, relaxed flow of energy. And depending on how you walk, it can be the precursor to a great night's sleep or a nap...or be a midday pick-me-up if your energy is flagging.

Do This:

Variation 1: Walk to sleep. If you're fatigued and planning to get some shut-eye, take yourself on a short to moderate-length walk first. Allow enough time afterwards for a brief cooldown period before you lie down.

On this kind of walk, the idea is to work up to a brisk pace fairly quickly...and follow that with a long, slow taper-down. This tends to burn off any remaining stress energy and then let you sink into "mellow mode"—preparing you for sleep.

→ Choose two routes—one that will take 15 minutes to walk, and one that will take 25 to 30 minutes. Also allow a minimum of 5 minutes at the end for cooldown. Depending on conditions—including weather, light or darkness, and how tired you are—this will give you a choice. Make sure both routes are relatively flat.

→ Set out walking at a *moderate pace* for the first *2 to 3 minutes.*

→ When you feel your heart and breathing rate adjusting to your pace...increase to a *more rapid pace* for *2 to 3 more minutes.* You may want to walk at a *brisk pace* until you feel yourself getting tired. Or, after *6 to 8 minutes...*

→ Start to gear down...returning to your *moderate pace* for *2 or 3 minutes.*

→ Every minute thereafter, *slow your pace slightly*...until you are down to a *slow walk* (think "window-shopping"). Remember your *5-minute* cooldown.

Variation 2: Walk to wake. Sometimes we hit the middle of the day never having gotten our metabolism "up and running"—so we're fatigued by stored stress, not genuinely tired because we've spent all our energy. This is when "walk to wake" can work.

On this kind of walk, you want to build up more gradually to a brisk pace...have a shorter taper-down at the end...and, of course, a 5-minute cooldown.

→ Choose your routes. They can be a little more challenging...because you *want* to kick your metabolism into a higher gear.

→ Set out walking at a *slower pace* for the first *2 to 3 minutes.*

→ Increase to a *moderate pace* for the next *2 to 3 minutes.*

→ Increase again to a *brisk pace.* You want to break a "light sweat."

→ Allow time for a *2- to 3-minute taper* to your original slower pace, followed by the same *5-minute slow walk* at the end to let yourself cool down.

This kind of walk can set your metabolism on a higher notch, generating enough energy to carry you for several hours. (It can also give you a break from mental tensions—an added benefit when stress-thinking or stressful conditions are robbing you of your energy!)

Strategy #3: Non-Impact Aerobics

If you can sneak a little bit of energizing exercise into your schedule, try Non-Impact Aerobics (NIA).*

NIA offers a metabolism-boosting workout without the pounding, draining intensity of high-impact aerobics. The routines are a blend of stretching, gentler and more fluid motions, and proper deep breathing. The emphasis is on "right form" and graceful movement—which helps you focus and achieve a wonderfully refreshing state of clear-mindedness.

---

* Also see the sidebar on page 87—"Pilates and Yoga."

Depending where you are in your personal energy cycle, NIA can give you a needed boost to energize you for the rest of the day…or burn off stress fatigue and prepare you for a great rest.

→ Check with your local community centers, gyms, and health clubs to sign up for NIA or similar exercise classes.

→ Purchase a videotape or DVD version of an NIA workout. These are available in many larger bookstores and through on-line book and tape dealers.

THE CAPACITY-BUILDING STRATEGIES (EXERCISE)

Strategy #4: Run for Your Life… or at Least Walk Fast

Running and fast walking both offer a tremendous range of benefits. Not only do they help balance your energy levels, they benefit your heart muscle and circulatory system, help reduce cholesterol, help regulate hormone production, and aid in weight control. They can also improve your social life if you join a running group or walk with friends…and boost your spirit if you pray or meditate while you're out there "truckin'."

If you're going to make running or fast walking one of your basic health strategies, here's what you can do to get the most benefit from your time in motion.

Do This:

Step 1: Purchase a heart-rate monitor. You'll need to get your heart rate up into what's called the "aerobic zone." This is the zone where your heart is pumping fantastic amounts of newly oxygenated blood (because of all that good deep breathing you're doing) through your body.

Step 2: Know your "aerobic zone"…and get into it for *at least 30 minutes three times a week.* Here's a chart to help you:

Age	Range
25	120 to 156 beats per minute
35	114 to 150 beats per minute
45	108 to 138 beats per minute
55	96 to 126 beats per minute

Certain health conditions may affect your heart rate and rhythm, so you should consult a doctor before embarking on an exercise routine.

Step 3: Stay *in* the "aerobic zone" and don't go above it. If increasing your heart rate *this* much is good, then making it beat even faster is better—right? *Wrong.* Above the "aerobic zone" is your "cardio zone." If you're an athlete in training, you'll want to know when to push into this zone and how long you can stay there—because it's the zone where you're putting a huge energy demand on your body and your efforts are starting to burn the glycogen stored in your muscles…which is just before you start to metabolize your muscle tissue. (This triggers *autocannibalism*, so you obviously don't want to stay in this zone for long.)

If you want to increase your energy, feel more "up," and have endurance…you can do so simply by training your body to stay in the "aerobic zone" for longer periods of time. (You'll also like the fat-burning benefits of this!)

Step 4: Eat a light meal or snack consisting mainly of complex carbohydrates about an hour *before* you run or fast-walk. This will give you the ready energy your body needs for fuel while you're in motion…*and* keep your stomach from grumbling that you're ignoring its needs while having yourself a jolly good time.

Step 5: Eat a light meal, in a 30-40-30 balance, about 30 minutes to an hour *after* your run or walk. This will replenish the energy supply in your bloodstream, begin to restore any glycogen you've used from your muscles, and begin to build new muscle tissue… because those muscle cells you've just pushed are going to be saying, "We need some help here. We're calling in reinforcements."

A good regimen of running or fast walking will build those long, sinewy muscles filled with energy...and help you feel more alive, alert, and clearheaded.

Strategy #5: Weight-Resistance Workouts

No, you don't have to become a bodybuilder...smeared in oil and wearing one of those embarrassingly tiny pieces of Lycra. But you can increase your body's capacity to store energy by building *muscle*. And that means weight-resistance training—aka "lifting."

Weight-resistance training can include both calisthenics (push-ups, pull-ups, and so on) and working out on weight machines or with dumbbells.

There are many routines you can use, and which one you use depends on your goals. Lifting lighter weights with more repetitions will give you long, sinewy muscles. Lifting heavier weights with fewer repetitions will give you thicker, knottier muscles.

More importantly, in terms of personal energy production, weight-resistance training

→ causes your muscles to send signals to your body that more muscle-tissue is needed to do the work you're asking them to do...

→ thus, creating more muscle cells full of healthy nutrient-energy, and

→ reducing stores of fat that cause you to feel sluggish.

Here Is Some Good General Advice:

1. Work with a trainer. You can find trainers at health clubs and rec centers. Make sure yours is certified. A good trainer will help you put together a routine appropriate for your current strength level and goals.

2. "Easy does it" is the best rule of thumb when you're beginning a weight-lifting routine or restarting one after more than six months away from the machines. Too many of us try to build too fast, lift too much weight, push too hard…and we cause ourselves serious injury. Plan to build slowly.

3. Eat properly before and after workouts. About an hour before a workout you should eat a meal consisting mainly of complex carbohydrates to fuel you up. About 30 minutes after a workout you should eat a snack, again consisting mainly of complex carbohydrates, to replace the readily-available energy for your blood to circulate. And about 60 minutes after a workout you should eat good proteins to help strengthen those muscles that are primed and ready to build more tissue.

More muscle will give you more energy—not only in terms of strength but also endurance. And the increase in your metabolic rate will leave you clearheaded…and ready to take on the rest of the day.

7

Energizing Tonics from Nature

B ack to those ads we mentioned in the opening chapter—the ones that say, "Take [this product] and experience personal energy that's somewhere close to nuclear fission."

Thanks to these ads, in part, our thinking about supplements has changed. We're starting to think of them as in the same category as food. Maybe this is because we now have food products that advertise the supplements they contain ("the Energy Sports Drink with *Ginseng!*"). But supplements are *not* food. And most of these products are disappointing at best. At worst, some are not even good for you. True, some may deliver a rush of energy, but as soon as the "instant lift" passes, your energy level usually drops like a stone.

The "instant energy" products—whether in pill or food form— should not be lumped into the same category as legitimate natural supplements that have a proven tonic effect.

Some Very Good Reasons for Using Natural Supplements

"Supplements" are what we need when we are not getting all of our nutrients from food. As we noted in the chapter on nutrition, it's best to get all your nutrients from whole-food sources. As is true with every ideal, however, this is not always practical or possible.

For a variety of reasons, many of us simply rely on processed foods that are found in the average grocery store. Whole foods have a much shorter shelf life, and maybe we just don't have the time to shop that frequently…or we don't have access to stores that sell fresh, whole-food products. "Fresh" and "all natural" foods are also pricey. Sometimes you just have to choose the "Feed-a-Hoard Family Pack" of chicken over the "all natural" thing in the next cooler rack that's the size of a sparrow.

Likewise, many of us travel for business—or we live life "on the fly"—and the "best" food choices aren't exactly available. Or our digestion has been "off"...or...or...the fact is, sometimes we just don't eat right. And at other times our bodies are just not able to absorb all the vitalizing nutrients we need.

Most of us can benefit from the proven tonic effects certain supplements provide.

When Should You Consider Taking Supplements for More Energy?

1. **Temporarily—when you've slipped into poor eating habits**...and you're filling in nutritional "gaps" while you're correcting your diet but still feeling sluggish.

2. **When you've been under stress**...because of emotional strains like nervous tension, depression, or anxiety, and feel down or depleted.

3. **When your sleep patterns are interrupted or changed.**

4. **When you've put a heavier workload on your body—** because of increased sports activity, childbearing or child care, or plain old hard work—and find yourself dragging.

5. **When sudden illness has wiped you out, or when you're dealing with a long-term condition** that's drained your energy resources.

6. **To boost your base-level metabolism** when you've been experiencing sluggish digestion or that "tired all the time" feeling.

Bottom line: While it's better to rely on food for all your nutrients, natural supplements can be part of the whole-person health regimen to boost and re-energize you under certain unavoidable conditions.

SUPPLEMENTAL ENERGY FOR A BETTER WORKOUT

During workouts, we call upon our body to exert a great amount of extra energy. One way to actually see this in operation is to strap on a heart-rate monitor...and watch what happens when we go from, say, walking on a level surface to climbing a hill. Our pulse can zoom up 10, 20, or 30 points in, almost literally, a heartbeat.

Some of us ignore our body's energy needs during a workout, wind up exhausted and sore, and mutter, "I'll never do *that* again." Others are into the old simplistic formula: "Consume carbohydrates before and protein after."

But the fact is, if you work out regularly for more than 45 minutes at a time and with intensity, you will deplete the energy-supplying nutrients that are circulating in your bloodstream...and then begin to drain the glycogen from your muscles. As a result, you will experience deep-body fatigue, more muscle soreness, and inflammation. *And*, as mentioned earlier, if you work out intensely for a long period of time you'll actually begin metabolizing your own muscles—the condition of autocannibalism, which starving people experience.

To avoid running out of fuel...or worse yet, feeding on your own muscle tissue...you need to have a good "energy plan" in place. Besides good nutrition, that plan can also include the use of supplements that will keep you using the quickly available energy from your bloodstream.

Believe it or not, some trainers recommend that you use caffeine before a workout. If you don't like caffeine, here are supplements you may want to try, so you can see which ones keep you energized best:

guarana	*L-creatine*
kava	*L-tyrosine*
kola nut	*L-phenylalanine*

For more specific information on these supplements, see below.

NATURAL ENERGIZERS
Herbal Tonics

- **Ginger.** Many of us know that ginger can settle an upset stomach—which is why we sip ginger ale when our digestion is off or keep ginger snaps in the car to help the kids ward off motion sickness. But the fact is, ginger also increases your metabolism, giving you a subtle but definite energy boost that can last for several hours. It's also an effective digestive aid, which means it will help your body to better metabolize the nutrients from other foods. For this reason, many people use it regularly in cooking.

  A final important note: Ginger also contains *phenols,* compounds that are believed to help inhibit the growth of certain cancers—in particular, skin cancer.

- **Guarana.** This natural stimulant, which can be taken in capsule form, is also a mood lifter...and a far better choice than ephedra (see "Ephedra Warning" on the next page). Its energizing lift is two-and-a-half times more potent than the caffeine from coffee, tea, or soft drinks, and it can last for hours.

  You should avoid using guarana later in the day, as it can put you in opposition to your natural sleeping pattern, thereby defeating your purpose in taking it.

- **Guggul.** Thanks to the growing popularity of ayurveda, India's system of natural medicine, herbs like guggul are now becoming available here in the West. This is a whole-body tonic, an *adaptogen* that boosts the health of every major body system. (Adaptogens strengthen the immune, endocrine, and nervous system by increasing the body's ability to adapt to external and internal stress.) As is true with all adaptogens, the effects of guggul are experienced over time. A 14- to 30-day course is recommended, after which time you're most likely to feel the strong lift, brighter spirit, and greater mental clarity this herb offers.

EPHEDRA WARNING

~

Warnings about ephedra are everywhere these days. *Take them seriously.*

Ephedra is an herbal stimulant contained in many "quick energy" and "fast weight-loss" products. Often you find it in convenience stores—in products that promise to keep you awake on the highway. Sometimes it's sold under the name *ma huang.*

Ephedra hits the heart and respiratory system with a jolt more powerful than caffeine. That in itself makes it dangerous. While it's racing around your system, the effects on your whole body are just as bad. During the time it's juicing up your nervous system, making it operate on "high," it's also depleting other major systems of your body...setting you up for a big letdown when the effects wear off.

If you're thinking about using ephedra for energy or weight loss...*don't.* Other natural stimulants are safer and just as effective.

- **Kola nut.** The effect of this tropical seed is slightly more intense and longer-lasting than that of caffeine. It is more intense than guarana and can give you a rush of energy and, possibly, a mild tingling sensation.

  Be aware, though, that higher doses can have a reverse effect, pushing you through an "up" phase...then dropping you into "slowdown." As with any natural substance, you should start with a lower dose and work up.

  Kola nut can be found both in capsule and in extract forms.

- **Maté** works much like guarana and kola nut. Large amounts of maté can overstimulate you, however, causing insomnia. This is always to be avoided. It also has diuretic properties, so overuse can lead to dehydration.

Maté usually comes in loose-leaf or extract form, and can be taken as a tea.

- **Rhodiola** is one of the most potent of the natural adaptogens, and as such it supports the functioning of every major system of your body. Among its many benefits, rhodiola increases your resistance to physical, emotional, and chemical stressors, making it one of the best herbal supplements to take if you find yourself overwhelmed with too many responsibilities or too much work to do. It also increases the production of serotonin in the brain, causing you to experience a deep calm—which makes it an effective alternative to pharmaceuticals if you are experiencing chronic anxiety or panic attacks or both. Because all your energies are not being drained by nervous tension, you feel more energized—naturally.

  Rhodiola is available in capsules, tablets, and in a dried leaf form that makes a fragrant, energizing tea.

- **Siberian ginseng.** Another of the potent whole-body tonics, Siberian ginseng is well-known as an effective way to keep yourself boosted in the face of life's many energy demands. Among other things it helps keep the cardiovascular system strong and the blood pressure steady. Look for the scientific names of this herb—*Eleuthero* or *E. senticosus*—on the label because many substitutes and impostors are sometimes used in place of authentic Siberian ginseng.

  Though Siberian ginseng is not primarily a sleep aid, it also helps regulate our wake/rest cycle. It not only boosts energy while we're awake, it allows us to sleep more deeply and for longer periods of time...and thus awaken more refreshed.

  Siberian ginseng comes in capsules and extract. In root form it makes an excellent tea.

Sleep Aids

Maybe nighttime is a problem for you. Nerves, restlessness, or too many worries can cause us to toss and turn in bed. So can pain, indigestion, or illness. The result is a poor night's sleep…and fatigue or exhaustion the next day.

The following natural supplements are effective as relaxants. They can help you slip into deeply restful sleep and then allow you to wake refreshed, not "hung over," the next day…feeling naturally energized.

- **Skullcap.** European herbalists have used this wonderful herb for hundreds of years. It's a soothing sleep aid, and it also relieves headaches.

    Though you may not find this endearing, skullcap was called "mad-dog herb" in the seventeenth century because it was effective in calming animals with rabies. (Obviously, today's manufacturers offer skullcap packaged in much smaller doses than those used on animals.)

    Skullcap comes in extract and capsule forms.

    Note: Skullcap's sedative effects are strong, and you should not drive after taking this herb.

- **Valerian** naturally quiets the mind and calms the body, making it a potent sleep aid. Women whose sleep is made uneasy because of menstrual cramps benefit from its muscle-relaxing properties as well.

    Valerian is available in capsules and in extract form.

    Note: Valerian is known to react with barbiturates and should not be used if you are taking drugs from this family of medicines. If you are taking benzodiazepene drugs like Ativan, Valium, or Xanax you should not use this herb. It also affects the metabolism of Clozaril, Coumadin, Elavil, Haldol, Theo-Dur, Tofranil, Zyfol, and Zyprexa.

    Valerian should also not be used during pregnancy. And you should not drive immediately after using this herb.

A Brace of Energizing Vitamins

A deficiency of just about any vitamin can cause your energy levels to sag. For this reason you may want to maintain a base level of the major vitamins by taking a good multi. Here's what you should know.

- **Multivitamins** have their pluses and minuses. On the plus side, you are theoretically getting "something of everything" every day…especially since many multis also contain doses of important trace minerals. In this sense they're better than nothing. It's also easier for most of us to remember to take "one in the morning."

  On the minus side, however, multis are a sort of "buckshot" approach to taking vitamins. Again, better than nothing… and the scattershot will undoubtedly hit some of your needs. But you can be *very* deficient in certain vitamins and not be getting enough of them in your multi. On the other hand, you may get an overload of another vitamin or a trace mineral—and while this may not hurt you, it's a waste. And if you find that your energy level increases, you won't know exactly what did the trick. Finally, your once-a-day dose may be out of your system by late in the day when you most need the boost.

  In any case, if you're going to take multivitamins here are some steps for getting the greatest benefit.

Do This:

→ **Always take your vitamins with food**. Do not take them "in place of" a meal. Their purpose is mainly to help your cells absorb food energy.

→ **If you're taking *only* multivitamins, take more than one a day.** Don't take two at once. Take one with breakfast and one with dinner. Because most vitamins are water-soluble, such factors as stress, caffeine consumption, and the energy expense of a demanding day can wash vitamins right out of your system in a matter of hours.

A better approach is to build on the foundation of one multivitamin. Beyond that, the vitamins most likely to benefit your whole body—and therefore most likely to boost your energy—are these:

- **B-complex.** This family of vitamins is responsible for boosting the functioning of more systems of your body than any other. In fact, the B vitamins bring vitality to *every* system of your body. Ironically, they're quickly depleted from our bodies when we're overworked, stressed, depressed or anxious, or sick.

  Take a look at what each of the B vitamins does to energize you, and you'll understand why supplementation is important.

  —B_1 *(thiamine)* promotes clear thinking by improving brain functioning. Also improves circulation, digestion, and overall energy.

  —B_2 *(riboflavin)* stimulates the production of energizing and immune-boosting hormones and helps oxygenate blood by improving the production of red blood cells.

  —B_3 *(niacin)* increases the release of food energy to the cells, cleans out toxins that make the blood sluggish, and controls cholesterol.

  —B_5 *(pantothenic acid)* assists in the production of hormones and red blood cells, and in the body's manufacturing of vitamin D.

  —B_6 *(pyroxodine)* assists in the production of enzymes, hormones, and proteins, and lowers homocysteine levels in your blood (elevated homocysteine being associated with confused thinking—even stroke and Alzheimer's disease).

  —B_7 *(biotin)* improves the release of energy from carbohydrates—a main source of available food energy.

  —B_9 *(folic acid)* lowers homocysteine levels and helps prevent birth defects.

  —B_{12} *(cobalamin)* is vital for red blood cell and energy production.

- **Vitamin C** is commonly associated with boosting your immune system and preventing colds. In fact, scientific studies have proven its ability to boost overall vitality, especially in higher doses. It helps the adrenal gland produce hormones that energize your body and promotes a sense of overall well-being.

Vitamin C with bioflavonoids is recommended. If you take C in higher doses than the allowance recommended by the U.S. Food and Drug Administration, be sure to drink generous quantities of water—16 ounces with the dosage—or kidney stones can result.

BUT ARE MY SUPPLEMENTS ANY GOOD?

Those TV "news magazine" programs like to run exposés on natural-product manufacturers whose claims turn out to be bogus. Independent laboratories have sometimes tested herbal products and other natural supplements, only to discover they contain little or none of the substances named on the labels.

How can you know if you're getting what you pay for? And just as important, how can you know if what you're paying for is of good quality?

Here are two Web sites you can go to to check out the supplement manufacturers from whom you're buying:

- *Dietary Supplement Quality Initiative.* DSQI reviews supplements and makes its findings known to the public online at <www.dsqi.org>. If you can't find what you're looking for, you may wish to call them at (617) 734-4123.

- *ConsumerLab.Com.* Many independent labs buy supplements right off the shelves, just like you do, and test them for potency and purity. Their findings are posted at this site, and are free to you just through logging on.

Amino-Acid Power

Your body needs amino acids to build healthy cells and muscle tissues. Additionally, they promote healthy biochemical processes throughout your body. Amino-acid deficiency stresses the system, causing a physical "slump" that leaves you feeling bone-tired...and that can even lead to depression.

A caution: Remember, amino acids = protein. Too much protein can be toxic to the kidneys and liver. High-protein diets and the overuse of amino-acid supplements (for weight loss, musclebuilding, or more energy) can result in toxicity. If you use amino acids you should be careful to flush your system with water to prevent overtaxing your liver and kidneys.

- **Branch-chain amino acids.** Better muscle tone or more muscle leads to greater personal energy. Here's where branch-chain amino acids (BCAAs) come in. Aminos are essential for the formation of healthy body tissue. When we consume normal protein, the body breaks it down for use where it's specifically needed—for instance, for skin repair or organ-tissue replacement, or in the muscles.

  The BCAAs—valine, leucine, and isoleucine—are scientifically formulated in a configuration that is closest to the protein used in building muscle tissue. Therefore, more protein goes directly to toning and building muscle. As well, BCAAs are precursors to the amino acids glutamine and alanine, which comprise 60 percent of your skeletal system. For this reason, BCAAs can also be helpful in maintaining good bone density.

- **L-creatine** has become a favorite of bodybuilders and exercise enthusiasts, though its other benefits lie beyond aiding the impulse to muscle up or slim down. Creatine stimulates the brain's production and use of neurotransmitting chemicals. This helps produce clarity of thought and the efficient use of nutrients at the cellular level, thus bringing sharper mental focus and a deep-down sense of being energized. Hence, it enhances workouts.

- **L-phenylalanine.** This amino acid can have noticeably stimulating effects almost immediately. At the same time, it creates a sense of "peace" and well-being because it stimulates the production of endorphins and serotonin. Its greatest benefits, however, are felt over time.

  Caution: Do not use phenylalanine if you suffer from anxiety or panic attacks, as it can intensify your condition. Never exceed the manufacturer's recommended dose of phenylalanine, because it is easy to abuse.

- **L-tyrosine** is much like phenylalanine in that its energy-boosting effects can be felt quickly. It also works by boosting the production of the brain's neurotransmitters.

  Warning: Do not use tyrosine if you are taking an antidepressant of the MAO-inhibitor type.

In Closing

The right supplements can improve your level of vitality. And of course, you will increase their energizing potency greatly when you combine them with a good diet and the exercise that fits with your lifestyle.

Now, as we come to the close of this book, we're going to shift focus briefly—from the details of personal energy creation to a broader view of where personal energy comes from.

In the section that follows—"Living In-Flow"—you'll find encouragement to make the single most important change anyone can make in order to have the most vital and exciting experience of *life* possible.

A Final Word:
Living In-Flow

There is one more thing you can do to have all the energy you need. In fact, it's possibly the *most important* thing you can do. If you use any combination of strategies in this book, while you'll have more energy than you have now, there's a more fundamental change you can make. And like nothing else, it can allow you to experience the most amazing energy.

I am referring to the need each one of us has to learn the great art of what might be called *living in-flow.*

Living in-flow is a term that describes that deep-current sense of *life* we experience in those moments...all too rare for most of us...when some amazing balance is struck—and all the energies of body, mind, and soul focus and move as one. We sense that *this* is the right place and the right time, and that in *this* moment we are in right relationship with ourselves, God, and the world. What we're doing at that moment is flooding our whole being with a deep sense of joy that makes the pieces of who we are fall into place...a deep sense of joy that "makes sense of us."

We may be taking on a titanic project and sweating our brains out...taking charge in the midst of an emergency...finding the missing piece that solves a complicated problem...clarifying someone's confusion...standing up for an underdog...offering a simple service that makes someone's life easier or more gracious...or standing motionless, totally focused, peering into the great beauty of some small natural wonder. In these moments, it's as if a fine current of the life energy that flows from the very Spirit of our Creator

107

is rushing from deep inside our spirit, through our heart and mind, and into our physical being…and we feel joyful satisfaction.

After experiencing such moments, people say things like, "It didn't feel like I was living—it felt like I was *being lived.*" A sense of enlargement, expanded awareness, and deep satisfaction in living has flooded us to the very nerve endings and made us realize, "This is what I need more of—and more often—in order to be who I am."

Is anything more energizing than finding the life we were meant to live? No wonder we experience a heightened sense of energy. In the Christian tradition, we look back to our Hebrew roots for an understanding, not only of the Source of all life collectively but the Source of our individual lives. How do I find *my* life—the life that gives me joy and purpose?

In the highly personal dialogues between the psalmist's deep soul and the One who is the giver of life, we find a clue to our own answer:

> *"You created my inmost being…*
> *I am fearfully and wonderfully made."*

When the psalmist speaks about his "inmost being," he's referring to the original spark of life ignited within him that gives him all the energies that make up an individual life—his essential self with all the passions, curiosities, interests, drives, and loves that make him *him.* The Hebrews believed that this spark was the gift of God to every soul created, making each one of us unique in all creation. The great challenge, they also recognized, was to use this passion in a way that was both self-expressing and also for the benefit of all—since life is a gift from the God who loves all—and not in purely selfish or destructive ways. As the great teacher Moses Maimonides put it, "If I am not for me, then who is for me? And if I am only for me, then what am I?"

Hebrew wisdom teaches us that finding the greatest, most energizing expression of who we are comes as we set out on a spiritual journey—first, to experience the passionate energies that are our soul…and then to find out how we can help this world and the other people in it with the energies that pour through us. This, for the believing person, offers a good understanding of what it ultimately means to live in-flow.

As well…it offers a beginning step and a challenge. We can hear a voice speaking out of the center of our restless discontent and all our dreams and yearnings:

"Before you were born, I breathed into you the creative fire of who you are. I made you, *you*—exactly as you are. I formed you and called you *good*. And I delivered you into a world where you are needed to make things better. Now what will you do with who you were made to be?"

Because you are uniquely created, *no one*, ultimately, can tell you how to live in-flow with who you are. God, it seems, has made us so individual that experiencing the divinely energetic ignition of *life* does not come about in exactly the same way for any two people.

What we do need, every one of us, is the courage to enter into that journey. To our rote faith—that is, the tenets we cling to—we need to add a spiritually energizing kind of faith. Faith to set out on the quest. Faith to believe that we can, we *need* to, move beyond the barriers that seem to keep us from living life in a deeper, more meaningful way. Faith that, as we struggle and face challenges, setbacks, even perhaps the misunderstanding and disapproval of other people, we are on the journey we are supposed to be on: the great adventure of living the life we were created to live.

Nothing is more wonderfully energizing.

In closing, I wish you a good journey. May you bravely face the choices and changes you may need to make to find the life of vitality, enthusiasm, passion, and meaning that is yours.

The New Nature Institute

The New Nature Institute was founded in 1999 for the purpose of exploring the connection between personal health and wellness and spirituality, with the Hebrew-Christian tradition as its spiritual foundation.

Drawing upon this tradition, the Institute supports the belief that humankind is created in the image of God. We are each body, mind, and spirit, and so intricately connected that each aspect of our being affects the others. If one aspect suffers, our whole being suffers; if all aspects are being supported, we will enjoy a greater sense of well-being.

For this reason, the Institute engages in ongoing research in order to provide up-to-date information that supports a "whole person" approach to wellness. Most especially, research is focused on the natural approaches to wellness that support health and vitality in the body, mind, and spirit.

Healthy Body, Healthy Soul is a series of books intended to complement treatment plans provided by healthcare professionals. They are not meant to be used in place of professional consultations and/or treatment plans.

Along with creating written materials, the New Nature Institute also presents seminars, workshops, and retreats on a range of topics relating to spirituality and wellness. These can be tailored for corporate, spiritual community, or general community settings.

For information contact:

David Hazard
The New Nature Institute
P.O. Box 568
Round Hill, Virginia 20142

(540) 338-7032
Exangelos@aol.com

Books by David Hazard in the Healthy Body, Healthy Soul Series

BREAKING FREE FROM DEPRESSION
Life is good. Don't lose any more time to crippling depression.

BUILDING CANCER RESISTANCE
Simple ways to boost your immune system's resistance to cancer.

OVERCOMING ANXIETY
Excellent strategies to help manage life-limiting fears.

REDUCING STRESS
Simple techniques to reduce stress—from relaxation to herbal teas.

TIRED NO MORE!
Natural energy-boosting strategies to restore vitality and joy to life.